Clinical Perspectives on Psychotherapy Supervision

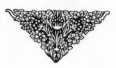

Edited by

Stanley E. Greben, M.D., F.R.C.P.C., F.R.C.Psych.

Professor Emeritus, Department of Psychiatry,
University of Toronto; Consultant,
Department of Psychiatry, Mount Sinai Hospital,
Toronto, Ontario, Canada

Ronald Ruskin, M.D., Dip. Psych., F.R.C.P.C.

Assistant Professor, Department of Psychiatry, and
Senior Research Associate, Trinity College,
University of Toronto; Staff Psychiatrist,
Mount Sinai Hospital, Toronto,
Ontario, Canada

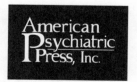

American
Psychiatric
Press, Inc.

Washington, DC
London, England

Note: The authors have worked to ensure that all information in this book concerning drug dosages, schedules, and routes of administration is accurate as of the time of publication and consistent with standards set by the U.S. Food and Drug Administration and the general medical community. As medical research and practice advance, however, therapeutic standards may change. For this reason and because human and mechanical errors sometimes occur, we recommend that readers follow the advice of a physician who is directly involved in their care or the care of a member of their family.

Books published by the American Psychiatric Press, Inc., represent the views and opinions of the individual authors and do not necessarily represent the policies and opinions of the Press of the American Psychiatric Association.

Copyright © 1994 American Psychiatric Press, Inc.
ALL RIGHTS RESERVED
Manufactured in the United States of America on acid-free paper
97 96 95 94   4 3 2 1
First Edition
American Psychiatric Press, Inc.
1400 K Street, N.W., Washington, DC 20005

Library of Congress Cataloging-in-Publication Data
Clinical perspectives on psychotherapy supervision / editors, Stanley
  E. Greben & Ronald Ruskin.
     p.   cm.
  Includes bibliographical references and index.
  ISBN 0-88048-552-3
  1. Psychotherapists—Supervision of.   I. Greben, Stanley E.
II. Ruskin, Ronald, 1944–   .
  [DNLM: 1. Psychotherapy–education. 2. Internship and Residency.
3. Mentors.   WM 19.5 C6413 1994]
RC459.C57   1994
616.89′023—dc20
DNLM/DLC
for Library of Congress   93-44802
                                                                        CIP

British Library Cataloguing in Publication Data
A CIP record is available from the British Library.

Contents

Contributors   vii

Foreword   xi
    Robert Michels, M.D.

**1   Introduction: Significant Aspects of the Supervisor-
Supervisee Relationship and Interaction**   1
    Stanley E. Greben, M.D., F.R.C.P.C.
    Ronald Ruskin, M.D., F.R.C.P.C.

**2   Ethical and Legal Issues in Psychotherapy
Supervision**   11
    Alan A. Stone, M.D.

3   Gender Issues in Supervision   41
    Carol C. Nadelson, M.D.
    Catherine Belitsky, M.D., F.R.C.P.C.
    Mary V. Seeman, M.D., F.R.C.P.C.
    Keith Ablow, M.D.

**4   Issues in Psychotherapy Supervision When
Participants Are From Different Cultures**   53
    Ronald Ruskin, M.D., F.R.C.P.C.

**5   Supervision of the Beginning Psychiatric
Resident**   73
    Stefan P. Stein, M.D.

6   The Supervisee's Experience of Supervision   85
    Jon Hunter, M.D., F.R.C.P.C.
    Debra A. Pinsky, M.D.

7   Supervision of Group Psychotherapy   99
    Molyn Leszcz, M.D., F.R.C.P.C.
    Leo Murphy, M.D., F.R.C.P.C.

8 Family Therapy Supervision   121
Leopoldo Chagoya, M.D., F.R.C.P.C.
Kenneth Citron, M.D., F.R.C.P.C.

9 Supervision of Patients With Recurrent Psychosis   135
Mary V. Seeman, M.D., F.R.C.P.C.
Melvin Prosen, M.D., F.R.C.P.C.

10 Emergency and Crisis Psychotherapy Supervision   151
Rodney Slonim, M.D., F.R.C.P.C.

11 A Cognitive-Behavioral Model of Supervision With Individual and Group Components   165
Marsha M. Linehan, Ph.D.
Debbie E. McGhee, B.A.

12 The Development of a Psychotherapy Supervisor   189
Leopoldo Chagoya, M.D., F.R.C.P.C.
Charlotte Chagoya, R.N., PG Psych. Nurs.,
Dip.Fam.Ther.

13 Privacy Versus Disclosure in Psychotherapy Supervision   211
Elizabeth Wallace, M.D., F.R.C.P.C.
Anne Alonso, Ph.D.

14 When Supervision May Fail: Difficulties and Impasses   231
Ronald Ruskin, M.D., F.R.C.P.C.

Index   263

Contributors

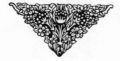

Keith Ablow, M.D.
Associate Medical Director, Tri-City Mental Health and Retardation
Center, Lynn, Massachusetts

Anne Alonso, Ph.D.
Associate Clinical Professor of Psychology, Department of
Psychiatry, Harvard Medical School, Cambridge, Massachusetts

Catherine Belitsky, M.D., F.R.C.P.C.
Fellow in Psychiatry, University of Toronto; Fellow, Clarke
Institute of Psychiatry, and Toronto Hospital, Toronto, Ontario,
Canada

Charlotte Chagoya, R.N., PG Psych. Nurs., Dip.Fam.Ther.
Lecturer, Department of Psychiatry, University of Toronto;
Coordinator, Couple/Family Therapy Program, Psychiatric Clinic
for HIV-Related Concerns, Mount Sinai Hospital, Toronto, Ontario,
Canada

Leopoldo Chagoya, M.D., F.R.C.P.C.
Associate Professor, Department of Psychiatry, University of
Toronto; Staff Psychiatrist and Head, Psychiatric Couple/Family
Therapy Clinic, Mount Sinai Hospital, Toronto, Ontario, Canada

Kenneth R. Citron, M.D., C.C.F.P., F.R.C.P.C.
Lecturer, Department of Psychiatry, University of Toronto; Staff
Psychiatrist, Mount Sinai Hospital, Toronto, Ontario, Canada

Stanley E. Greben, M.D., F.R.C.P.C., F.R.C.Psych.
Professor Emeritus, Department of Psychiatry, University of
Toronto; Consultant, Department of Psychiatry, Mount Sinai
Hospital, Toronto, Ontario, Canada

Jon Hunter, M.D., F.R.C.P.C.
Assistant Professor, Department of Psychiatry, University of Toronto; Staff Psychiatrist and Head, Psychosomatic Service, Mount Sinai Hospital, Toronto, Ontario, Canada

Molyn Leszcz, M.D., F.R.C.P.C.
Associate Professor and Head, Psychotherapy Program, Department of Psychiatry, University of Toronto; Staff Psychiatrist and Head, Group Therapy Service, Mount Sinai Hospital, Toronto, Ontario, Canada

Marsha M. Linehan, Ph.D.
Professor of Psychology and Adjunct Professor of Psychiatry and Behavioral Sciences; Director, Suicidal Behaviors Research Clinic, University of Washington, Seattle, Washington

Debbie E. McGhee, B.A.
Clinical Psychology Graduate Student, University of Washington, Seattle, Washington

Robert Michels, M.D.
The Stephen and Suzanne Weis Dean and Barklie McKee Henry Professor of Psychiatry, Cornell University Medical College, New York, New York

Leo Murphy, M.D., F.R.C.P.C.
Assistant Professor, Department of Psychiatry, University of Toronto; Staff Psychiatrist and Head, Psychiatric Outpatient Services, St. Michael's Hospital, Toronto, Ontario, Canada

Carol C. Nadelson, M.D.
Professor, Department of Psychiatry, Tufts University School of Medicine, Boston, Massachusetts; Staff Psychiatrist, Cambridge Hospital, Cambridge, Massachusetts

Debra A. Pinsky, M.D.
Clinical Associate, Experimental Therapeutics Branch, National Institute of Mental Health, Bethesda, Maryland

Melvin Prosen, M.D., F.R.C.P.C.
Staff Psychiatrist, Sheppard and Enoch Pratt Hospital, Towson, Maryland (deceased)

Ronald Ruskin, M.D., Dip. Psych., F.R.C.P.C.
Assistant Professor, Department of Psychiatry, and Senior Research Associate, Trinity College, University of Toronto; Staff Psychiatrist, Mount Sinai Hospital, Toronto, Ontario, Canada

Mary V. Seeman, M.D., F.R.C.P.C.
Professor and Vice-Chair, and Head, Schizophrenia Program, Department of Psychiatry, University of Toronto; Head, Schizophrenia Program, Clarke Institute of Psychiatry, Toronto, Ontario, Canada

Rodney Slonim, M.D., F.R.C.P.C.
Assistant Professor, Department of Psychiatry, University of Toronto; Staff Psychiatrist and Head, Psychiatric Emergency and Crisis Intervention Service, Mount Sinai Hospital, Toronto, Ontario, Canada

Stefan P. Stein, M.D.
Professor of Clinical Psychiatry, Cornell University Medical College; Director of Residency Education, Payne Whitney Clinic, New York Hospital, New York, New York

Alan A. Stone, M.D.
Professor of Law and Psychiatry, Faculty of Law and Faculty of Medicine, Harvard University, Cambridge, Massachusetts

Elizabeth Wallace, M.D., F.R.C.P.C.
Lecturer, Department of Psychiatry, University of Toronto; Staff Psychiatrist, Mount Sinai Hospital, Toronto, Ontario, Canada

The editors are grateful to Tammy LePage for all of her help in the preparation of the original manuscript.

Foreword

Supervision is the central experience in becoming a psychotherapist. There are, of course, other essentials that are relevant—capacity or talent, professional socialization, and cognitive learning about psychology, psychopathology, psychodynamics, and theories of psychotherapy. However, psychotherapy is very much a *praxis,* a *doing,* rather than a *gnosis,* a *knowing*—a person only learns to do something by doing it. When that involves other people, their lives, their views of themselves, and their relationships with others, the student cannot just start by practicing. Too much is at stake, and the beginning therapist would find it impossible to be honest with the patient, to be honest with him- or herself, and to invite the patient into an unsupervised treatment new also to the therapist. As a result, supervision is not only central, it is necessary to the development of the psychotherapist.

Of course, supervision is helpful in the acquisition of other skills as well. However, it has a special relationship to psychotherapy, because in many respects, the supervisory process mirrors the therapeutic one. This mirroring offers interesting potentials—as in the exploitation of the parallelism as a window on the therapeutic relationship. But it also presents possible dangers—as in the frequent contamination of otherwise good supervision by inappropriate excursions into psychotherapy. The special relationship is also reflected by the common tendency to structure supervision so that it resembles the therapy being supervised (e.g., the use of group supervision for group psychotherapy).

There are, of course, important differences as well. The data on supervision are much more accessible than those of psychotherapy, and so it is easier to record, observe, share, and even supervise supervision than it is psychotherapy. In supervision, the domain of interest is more cognitive and less emotional, and most supervisees are less demanding than their patients. Supervision is also extraordinarily complex: the supervisor must take into account the patient, along with his or her pathology, dynamics, life situation, and treatment goals; the therapist, along with his or her stage of development, intellectual understanding, countertransferences, and career goals; and the therapeutic and supervisory processes and the professional and institutional contexts in which these all occur. Though it is impossible to be aware of all of these issues at one time, the well-trained supervisor understands them and has access to them when relevant.

This book is an immensely valuable resource for any supervisor who wants to be a good one, and for any supervisee who has had enough experience to be interested in the process. It examines supervision from multiple perspectives: type of therapy (group, family, behavioral, psychodynamic); type of patient (e.g., with a psychosis or in a crisis); context (legal, ethical, cultural, gender); vantage of the supervisee; development of the supervisor; and even from the perspective of failed supervision. The authors explore theory, review the literature, offer guidelines for practice, provide many useful clinical vignettes, and discuss the relevant empirical research.

If you are not a supervisor, reading this book will not make you one. But if you are a supervisor, it is certain to make you a better one. Drs. Greben and Ruskin have collected their own experience and that of their colleagues and have done an immense service to the profession in the process.

Robert Michels, M.D.

Chapter 1

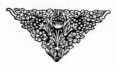

Introduction: Significant Aspects of the Supervisor-Supervisee Relationship and Interaction

Stanley E. Greben, M.D., F.R.C.P.C., and
Ronald Ruskin, M.D., F.R.C.P.C.

Our purpose in this book is to explore in detail various aspects of the supervision of psychotherapy. Behind this undertaking lies a set of general principles that have guided the collaboration that has produced this work.

First, we take the psychotherapies to be an essential, indigenous part of medicine, of psychiatry, and of other helping professions such as psychology and social work. In times when the pendulum of psychiatric thinking swings more toward the biological and away from the psychological, it is essential to remind ourselves that helping people can never be divorced from listening to and talking with them (Greben 1992).

Second, whereas it is clear that students of psychotherapy learn in a variety of ways, both intellectual and experiential, one of the most important ways of learning is through supervision of psychotherapy. Within the supervisory experience are numerous elements, and these

1

we will attempt to identify and elucidate.

Third, we wish to illustrate that psychotherapy supervision is, like psychotherapy itself, a highly personal undertaking on the parts of both the supervisor and the supervisee. It can take place between two individuals, among a group of professional peers, or it can be formal or informal. Yet it will always be a reflection of the attitudes, experience, and personalities of those people who participate in it.

Finally, we believe that when psychotherapy supervision maintains that highly individual flavor, it will be at its best. The chapters of this book illustrate that same principle, for each is an idiosyncratic expression, in the words of its author or authors, of one aspect of or one approach to supervision. We hope that, once all of these personal views and approaches have been read, there will emerge an integrated response within the reader, one that will further and deepen attitudes about this complex human endeavor. Should that be the case, our fundamental purpose will have been fulfilled.

The relationship between psychotherapy supervisor and supervisee can be best understood by comparing it to other traditional relationships in society. It is on the one hand a teacher-student relationship where objective knowledge is transmitted. On the other hand, it is a craftsman- or artisan-apprentice relationship, where subjective experience is discussed and shared. We explore some of the ramifications of these two types of working relationships.

There are some tasks that, when a person sets out to learn them, are so simple or so straightforward that he or she can simply be shown how to do them. An example would be the use of a simple tool, say a hammer or a key. There are other tasks that are much more complicated to perform and that also benefit from the personal variations in performance that are brought to the task. Psychotherapy falls in the latter category, not the former. Whereas there is a body of scientific knowledge and practical experience that can be passed on from the experienced practitioner to the trainee, the teaching-learning undertaking involves much more than that. As with most complex professional roles, learning to be a psychotherapist involves the development of the student's capacity to make moment-to-moment decisions and responses, as well as the growth of the student's self-confidence in the use of his or her own talents and personal attributes. The learning process should also provide for the student's growing sense of freedom of action—one that is not only based on the understanding of traditional methods and approaches, but that also fosters exploration as well as the freedom to learn from the clinical task at hand (see Chapter 14).

The student who has not been exposed to conventional approaches and to the historical context of the profession is ignorant in ways that will severely limit his or her ability to perform the work. On the other hand, the student who cannot move at all from the models and guides that have been put forward in training will be disabled in the opposite direction: he or she will have a series of preformed patterns from which to choose, but insufficient adaptive capacity to meet the wide variety of clinical challenges. The task of the teacher, and of the training program, is to encourage the student to avoid both of these restrictive extremes.

As we approach the 21st century, it would be ingenuous to suggest that the relationship between an individual who is teaching and one who is learning psychotherapy is uniquely different from roles that have existed through earlier centuries. Our task as educators is to try to recognize and identify the desired attributes of such a relationship, as well as the sound educational and interpersonal principles upon which they are based.

Let us first examine the task of transmitting facts or information that the teacher must undertake. There are many ways in which this takes place in psychotherapy supervision. The most important occurs when the supervisor says what he or she would do in a given situation, or what he or she has done in past similar situations. Of course a supervisor does not say, or even imply, "This is the way to do it." That would be acceptable for one of the two simple examples of using a hammer or a key, but it would not be appropriate for the complex role that we are attempting to teach. In saying, or implying, "This is what I would do," the supervisor is offering one approach for the supervisee to consider. The guidance is opening the supervisee's mind to a possible course of action, but he or she is only to follow that course if he or she feels it to be consistent with his or her own judgment and spontaneous inclinations.

The second way to impart information is to give clinical examples from the supervisor's own work (or from his or her own life experiences) to place options before the supervisee that may not otherwise occur to him or her. The third source of information is through the recommendation of publications that the supervisee might benefit from reading. These will ordinarily be writings that have had a positive helpful effect upon the teacher and that he or she thinks are illustrative of principles of which he or she wishes to make the student more aware. When the supervisor is someone who publishes papers on related subjects or conducts clinical research, it is opportune for him or her to present these to the student as more personal illustrations of his or her approach to psychotherapeutic work.

All of these examples of the presentation of information call for a democratic rather than an autocratic stance on the part of the supervisor. We are not discussing early education—we are discussing the highest level of postgraduate education. And we are doing so with students, many of whom have various undergraduate degrees, and all of whom have medical or other graduate degrees and who are in the course of speciality training. The wise teacher presents to such very senior students a selected variety of options, and, at the same time, offers the freedom of choosing from among them.

We have stated that the relationship between supervisor and supervisee has much in common with that of teacher and student, as well as with that of artisan and apprentice—relationships such as have existed through many centuries. Both these models require the transmission of information and of experience from the senior to the junior colleague. Yet they also require a great deal else, all the more so in the pursuit of a complex professional task such as psychotherapy. If a person is making ceramic pots or taking still life photographs, he or she may not need to learn how to relate to others in the course of doing the work. If a person is to shoe horses or to be a veterinarian, that person must certainly know how to relate to animals, for the perfect shoe does the horse no good until it has been affixed properly. If a person is to be a physician, or a portrait photographer, or an orchestra conductor or a psychotherapist, he or she must (while learning the facts of the profession) acquire the approaches and attitudes that allow a person to practice the art of the profession. It is difficult to imagine that anyone could expect to be competent in working closely or even intimately with other people and have no direction or assistance or guidance in what makes work with other people more likely to be successful. It is this second and major portion of the teaching responsibility of the psychotherapy supervision that we address next.

How do the teacher, the craftsman, the artisan, and the physician teach the ways in which to deal with students, clients, customers, or patients? Certainly not by ignoring the subject. Unfortunately, as physicians and as educators, we are often told by interested members of the public that we teach our students too successfully by poor example. They often ask medical educators how the brightest, most strongly motivated high school graduates can, in a few years' time, be so frequently converted to rather rude and apparently insensitive medical interns or residents. The answer does not appear to lie in the injudicious choice of candidates accepted into medical schools. Rather, it lies in the example set the medical students by their teachers: how they deal with students, with patients, and with colleagues. The same is the case for practitioners of other professions.

If that is so, then what does all this say for psychotherapy supervision? It says that the teacher is not only important for didactic purposes (i.e., as an instructor or informant) but also as an example and a guide. Supervisees learn much more from what supervisors do, or from what they say they would do or have done with patients, than from what theories they espouse (Greben 1991). That does not mean that supervisors need to be self-conscious about their behavior within supervisory sessions. On the contrary, they would best be spontaneous and natural, rather than awkward, contrived, or anonymous. This means that they must be aware of the complex ways in which a respected teacher influences the attitudes and behavior of a less experienced colleague. The supervisor should freely expose to the supervisee his or her views, doubts, concerns, guiding principles—and ignorance. Humility on the part of the teacher fosters both respect and humility on the part of a student. This approach will not be successful if it is based on artifice. The arrogant teacher with a falsely humble presentation will be recognized as such by the astute student. The teacher who knows how much he or she knows as well as how much he or she does not and cannot know inspires the student to maintain a skeptical attitude and an open-minded wish to learn.

How is this to be translated into activity on the part of the teacher? The teacher must listen a lot and tell the student what he or she thinks is being said. He or she must be cautious about how the student is criticized—not because the student should not become aware of the teacher's opinions, but because it is important to have the student feel safe and not threatened in the teacher's company. The supervisor is, after all, an experienced psychotherapist, as is (to a lesser extent) the supervisee. Each of them has to be adept at telling others—patients or clients—things that are uncomfortable to hear. At the same time, each of them should have learned that patience and tactfulness can bring important rewards to the therapist and, indeed, to anyone interested in being of psychological help to others. The impatient, grating supervisor will not encourage the awkward supervisee to seek his or her help. Rather, he or she will foster a greater degree of the nondisclosure that, under the best circumstances, occurs in all supervisory situations (see Chapter 13). Respectful comments by a concerned teacher will help the student become aware of his or her own insensitivities or blind spots, especially those of countertransference origin.

Tact and respectfulness still leave considerable room for honesty and candor on the part of the supervisor. What can be wrought through patient, understanding perseverance cannot be wrought through either silence or tough-minded confrontations (Chapter 6).

When conditions in the supervisory relationship are good enough, the supervisee will identify with the supervisor as one of his or her professional models. We say "one of," because it is highly desirable for the supervisee to have a number of such models. Building a professional identity occurs most readily when numerous models are available. There should be consecutive models (which the student has during the various years of his or her training) as well as concurrent models, so that the student can compare teachers who work with him or her during the same period. The good supervisor is respected but not held in awe. The student admires a competent, accomplished teacher but understands that there is more than one way to be a psychiatrist or psychotherapist, and more than one approach and attitude toward the practice of psychotherapy. The student understands that the teacher is implying: "Hear what I say and watch what I do; try it on for size, and do the same with your other supervisors. Keep what suits you and reject what does not. Remember what I have said and done, for sometime you may want to say and do the same. Learn from all your experiences; don't trust only what you have learned from your teachers. Someday, when you are the teacher, offer your students this same freedom; and also learn from your students, as I have learned from you."

> A resident came to her first psychotherapy supervision session with some apprehension. She was in the final 6 months of her psychiatric residency, and the patient she chose to present had been seen by her for 2½ years. She felt awkward, because she felt stuck: the psychotherapy seemed to have plateaued and had become stiff and boring.
>
> Within the first part of the supervisory hour, the supervisor felt that the resident had been inhibiting herself in an unnatural way. She appeared to be an emotionally warm and responsive person, yet she reported that she had felt constrained to be formal and anonymous with her female patient. The supervisor wondered if she might allow herself to be more forthcoming, answering some of the simple and valid questions that the patient had occasionally and hesitatingly put to her. This modest question allowed the resident to begin to be more open with her patient, disclosing material that was specific but not too highly personal.
>
> The work with her patient changed very markedly in the ensuing weeks and months: the patient was grateful for the trust and confidence the resident showed in her, and the resident felt relieved of her guilt that she had been unnaturally and uncharacteristically withholding.
>
> The supervisor's mild comment had allowed the resident to make a considerable shift in her approach to the patient, freeing the resident to be more responsive yet still highly professional.

The effective therapist helps his or her patients to learn a great deal. At the same time, such a therapist learns from every patient (Greben and Seeman, in press). Often he or she learns something new. At other times, the therapist confirms that what others have taught him or her is also true with the patient at hand. Just as every patient teaches every effective physician, every student teaches every effective supervisor. Supervisor and supervisee both recognize that one is the more experienced, that one is the guide and the other the follower. However, they should also acknowledge that in any teaching-learning experience, the teaching and the learning are in both directions.

To learn a craft, an art, a science, or a profession, a person must have an atmosphere that is free, relatively benign, emotionally supportive, scientifically inquiring, curious, positively skeptical, open-minded, accepting, and humane. Insofar as such an atmosphere exists in the supervisor-supervisee relationship, both will learn and, as a consequence, future patients and future generations of students will benefit. In the end, both supervisor and supervisee will carry away from their work together respect and gratitude for a helpful and rewarding collegial experience.

The Multifaceted Nature of the Supervisory Relationship

We have described some of the characteristics of the supervisor as teacher and model. In certain ways, as numerous authors have described, there are similarities between supervisory and therapeutic relationships. However, there are important differences. The supervisor comes to teach and to guide, not to treat. Nonetheless, there should be room within the supervisory relationship for comments that lead the supervisee to understand more about him- or herself. This is, after all, the case in all good didactic and training experiences: the student or trainee, while learning about the subject at hand, learns more about him- or herself.

There are times during supervision of psychotherapy when the supervisor feels free to point out to the supervisee some attitudes or practices that stand in the way of doing his or her best work. Considerable caution and careful judgment are necessary here so as not to switch to a therapeutic role. The supervisor is a professional who is very experienced in dealing with people. At times, he or she can bring additional benefit to the supervisee by pointing to personal difficulties that are reflected within the work they are discussing.

It is not the supervisor's task to identify the sources of these difficulties. However, he or she can make observations about what stands in the way of the work and indicate that the supervisee might find it helpful to further pursue understanding those difficulties within another (therapeutic) context. When, for example, the supervisee's manifest anxiety in his or her psychotherapeutic work is so great that it effectively inhibits any clinical progress or self-understanding, and supportive supervisory measures are unsuccessful in addressing the supervisee's recurrent therapeutic impasses, an honest and direct discussion of personal therapy may be indicated (Rubin 1989).

The supervisory relationship will also be influenced by the fact that, as is often the case in training programs, the teacher has not only a supervisory role but also an evaluative one. When the supervisee knows that he or she is to be judged or graded by the supervisor, he or she may withhold just those concerns or weaknesses that are most in need of supervisory attention. There is no way in which this conflict can be totally eliminated, for part of the teacher's role is to evaluate the student. However, the conflict can be diminished if within the supervisory relationship a supportive, encouraging, and helping atmosphere is fostered by the supervisor. This leads to an air of mutual trust, colleagueship, and collaboration, rather than one of contest, confrontation, and challenge. When such a positive atmosphere infuses the supervisory meeting, there is adequate room for the supervisor to make appraising, helpful comments to the supervisee—comments that can be received with respectful appreciation.

The supervisory relationship does not exist in a vacuum. Rather, it resides within an educational and administrative context. It can be helpful on occasion to turn to others within that context. The colleague who is in charge of postgraduate education can be most useful. At times, supervisor and supervisee can look for such assistance with awkward difficulties in the supervisee or supervisory relationship. The postgraduate education coordinator may be perceived as being more at arm's length and hence in a better position to respond objectively.

In summary, there will be times when personal difficulties intrude into the supervisor-supervisee relationship and when others need to be involved. In the large majority of instances, this is not the case. Rather, the "good enough" supervisory relationship will allow a mutually trusting and cooperative atmosphere to exist in the supervisory room, and whatever friction arises can be dealt with by the two participants.

Summary and Conclusions

The supervisor-supervisee relationship is a professional one that reflects the personalities, attitudes, and values of the two participants. It encompasses that of teacher-student, artisan-apprentice, and mentor-protégé. Because emotional and personal matters are being discussed, and because both participants are also at other times psychotherapists, both are aware of their personal contributions to their interactions. When both are successful in establishing an atmosphere of mutual trust and collaborative colleagueship, psychotherapy supervision can be helpful and rewarding to both participants and, indirectly, to the patients being treated by the supervisee.

We hope that the chapters that follow serve to enhance the likelihood that readers, whether in the role of supervisor or supervisee, will be successful in establishing such fruitful working relationships.

References

Greben SE: Interpersonal aspects of the supervision of individual psychotherapy. Am J Psychother 45:306–316, 1991

Greben SE: The place of psychotherapy in medicine and the related professions. Paper presented at the First International Study Day, Latner Institute for Research in Social Psychiatry and Psychotherapy, Jerusalem, Israel, November 1992

Greben SE, Seeman MV: Learning from the patient: a clinical and educational approach. Humane Medicine (in press)

Rubin SS: At the border of supervision: critical moments in psychotherapists' development. Am J Psychother 43:387–392, 1989

Chapter 2

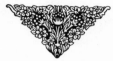

Ethical and Legal Issues in Psychotherapy Supervision

Alan A. Stone, M.D.

Psychotherapy Supervision: New Burdens and Risks

Psychotherapy supervision has rarely been the direct focus of judicial inquiry. Lawyers writing for the mental health professions have generally based their legal analysis on borrowed doctrines and case law related to other forms of supervision (Cohen and Mariano 1982; Slovenko 1980). Because so few cases have been decided by courts, authors have also relied on reports of cases settled out of court (Cohen and Mariano 1982), anecdotal accounts, and hypothetical cases (Slovenko 1980). Although the legal risks are great, the actual frequency of malpractice claims made against psychotherapy supervisors seems to have been less than anticipated. For example, "they account for only 9% of total malpractice claims" filed against psychologists (Austin et al. 1990). There is, in short, a very weak data base to justify the baleful warnings about the legal risks of psychotherapy supervision (e.g., "the greatest risk of liability" [Simon 1991]; the "suit of the future" [Slovenko 1980]). Whether or not these legal warnings were justified, they seem to have influenced the mental health professions to reevaluate the enterprise of psychotherapy supervision (Cormier et al. 1982; Harrar et al. 1990; Minnes 1987; Tanenbaum et al. 1990). As a result, the role of psychotherapy supervisor has taken on new legal and ethical dimensions (Harrar et al. 1990).

The nature of the change can be characterized as a shift from a simple to a complex paradigm. In the simple paradigm, the psychotherapy supervisor was an autonomous *consultant* who provided a hybrid, educational-therapeutic service to the supervisee (Ekstein and Wallerstein 1958). In the complex paradigm, the supervisor is presumed to have a primary responsibility for the patient (Austin et al. 1990; Harrar et al. 1990; Tanenbaum et al. 1990). He or she must also be aware of the conflicts in the administrative, educational, and therapeutic functions of the supervisory role. The supervisor must be prepared to monitor the clinical progress of the patient and, as steward and disciplinarian, report to the appropriate institutional authorities (Rinas and Clyne-Jackson 1988).

The legal and ethical considerations that have imposed these conflicting burdens on the supervisor are briefly outlined here to provide the reader with an initial overview.

First, the organizational structure of most hospitals, clinics, and other institutional health care providers has been drastically altered by law (Perkes 1986), regulation (Donaldson 1982, 1986), and managed care (Robiner et al. 1990). The locus of authority has moved from the individual attending staff members to the central administration. Centralized authority typically functions through committees (e.g., peer review, utilization review, risk management, etc.), and the supervisor is drawn into this bureaucracy. Even in private practice, managed care may have the authority to impose professional and economic constraints on psychotherapy, and therefore on supervision (Robiner et al. 1990).

Second, the real increase in malpractice claims against mental health professionals has (Austin et al. 1990) probably exposed supervision to new liability risks. Knowledgeable commentators have concluded that the psychotherapy supervisor is liable for his or her own negligent supervision and, even more importantly, may be vicariously liable for the negligence of the supervisee (Slovenko 1980).

Third, each of the mental health professions has strengthened and has begun to enforce its principles of ethics (Van Hoose and Kottler 1985). Institutions, such as hospitals and medical schools, and various boards of professional licensure have done the same (Cohen and Mariano 1982). This new enforcement is primarily directed at unethical clinical practice. However, the psychotherapy supervisor's ethical responsibilities have been redefined and the obligation to patients emphasized. The supervisor's relationship to the trainee has also been a target of criticism regarding abuses of power, sexual exploitation, and other conflicts of interest arising out of unethical "dual relationships" (Huber and Baruth 1987).

Fourth, psychotherapy supervision had been used to generate third-party payment in a deceptive entrepreneurial manner (Slovenko 1980) analogous to ghost surgery. The supervisor, typically a psychiatrist, billed the third-party payer for therapy actually performed by trainees or by other mental health professionals who were not authorized providers. Alternatively, supervisors who provided little or no supervision signed off on bills so that third-party payment could be obtained by otherwise nonqualified providers. These entrepreneurial arrangements were often unethical, if not actually fraudulent and illegal. There were a variety of legal and professional responses to "ghost supervision." Slovenko warned that the entrepreneurial psychiatrist would be vicariously liable for his or her enterprise and all of the patients who were supposedly treated. The various guilds took official positions and revised their codes of ethics to assert their independence. These professional posturings fostered the legal notion that the supervisor was responsible for the supervisee's patients. Billing practices are now carefully regulated; abuses can lead to punitive civil and criminal sanctions (Cohen and Mariano 1982). "Marketplace" practices continue to pose ethical and legal problems as psychotherapists compete for remuneration.

These and other developments have had certain common consequences. The enterprise of psychotherapy supervision is increasingly subject to private and public regulation and oversight. What was once another kind of teaching relationship is now encumbered by bureaucratic constraints, conflicting responsibilities, and legal liabilities.

The paradigm of psychotherapy supervisor has also been complicated by developments within the field of psychotherapy and psychotherapy training. Three themes frequently found in the supervision literature that are also particularly relevant to legal and ethical issues are discussed here (Loganbill et al. 1982): 1) drawing the line between supervision and treatment (Burns and Holloway 1989), 2) video technology and the closed-door model of supervision (Schlessinger 1966), and 3) the waning of dynamic psychotherapy and the identity crisis of supervision (Loganbill et al. 1982). These phases correspond roughly to the periods pre–World War II, post–World War II, and in more recent times.

Supervision or Therapy

Early in the history of psychoanalysis, when psychotherapy supervision became a central feature of training (Hess 1980), supervision focused on the trainee's own neurosis and his or her countertransference and its unconscious components. Freud had commented, "We have noticed that every analyst's achievement is limited by what his own complexes and resistances permit." The pedagogical task for the supervisor was to uncover the supervisee's unconscious complexes, resistances, and countertransference and alter them. The classic psychoanalytic solution would involve free association (DeBell 1963).

Some training institutes tried to solve the pedagogical task by having the training analyst also serve as the supervisor of the first analytic case while the trainee continued his or her own analysis (DeBell 1963). This arrangement, which called on the analyst to take on an additional and different role, complicated the trainee's transference and the termination, both crucial aspects of the analytic process. Other training institutes solved the problem by assigning another psychoanalyst as the supervisor. But in this novel approach, the supervisor would put the trainee on the couch and have him or her free-associate about the case. This so-called "Hungarian" method opened the door to the unconscious in quite unpredictable ways and tended to produce even more uncertainty about the supposed boundary between analysis and supervision.

Eventually, analytic training was organized so that students would begin to analyze patients during their own training analysis. However, a trainee would be assigned a separate supervisor for the case. In theory, this provided the trainee with the opportunity to free-associate about his or her case with the training analyst in order to explore his or her own limiting complexes and resistances as an analyst, while supervision was limited to face-to-face discussions and did not encourage or require free association (Langs 1980).

This arrangement, which became standard practice, established a boundary between analytic supervision and treatment. The supervisee would not be asked to free-associate. The supervisor was not expected to focus on the supervisee's unconscious or intimate fantasy life even when it touched on his or her analytic work, because that would take place in the training analysis. The supervisor was not there to analyze the trainee or to provide therapy; supervision was to be something else.

The boundary was not clearly demarcated. Certainly, many supervisors established a supportive if not an interpretive therapeutic relationship with the supervisee as they discussed technique, transference, and tactics. But the supervisee's "complexes and resistances" that concerned Freud were not to be grist for the mill of supervision.

This example of the beginnings of psychoanalytic supervision is of more than historical significance. Psychoanalysts believe that the training analysis is the most important learning experience in the process of becoming a psychoanalytic psychotherapist. Supervision is an important supplement but does not substitute for the experience of being a patient, or for the opportunity to achieve self-understanding. These experiences are only available during the trainee's own analysis. Traditional psychoanalytic training could theoretically draw a clear line between supervision and treatment, because the necessary treatment was going on elsewhere.

Many other psychotherapy training programs continue to focus on the importance of the learning experience of being a patient (Loganbill et al. 1982) but do not provide such an experience. They have continued to struggle with what is now called the "dual relationship" of supervisor and therapist, which has become a subject of serious pedagogical and ethical dispute. Many writers on psychotherapy supervision have considered the process a kind of intermediate or partial therapy and therefore inherently a dual relationship (Loganbill et al. 1982). A survey of psychodynamic supervision described two extremes. At one extreme, supervision focuses on the needs and problems of the trainee's patient; at the other, on the trainee's problems in relation to the patient, and even on the trainee's transference to the supervisor (Nemiah 1971). It is difficult to imagine how a dual relationship could possibly be avoided at the latter extreme.

The historical "Hungarian" detour in which the psychoanalytic supervisor asked the trainee to free-associate is also instructive. The method of psychoanalysis—free association—was thought to be essential to supervision. Similarly, as new schools of psychotherapy have emerged, their methods of supervision have often been an analogue or homologue to their methods of therapy (Hess 1980). The method of therapy is typically based on that school's theory of how psychological learning best takes place (Blocher 1983). The nondirective therapy of Carl Rogers and his nondirective supervision and experience-based learning provide one of the most compelling illustrations (Rogers 1980). From a quite different orientation, behavioral psychotherapists consider it theoretically possible to distinguish between the methods of therapy and supervision, but in practice they find no distinction (Hess 1980).

Thus, whatever the ethical guidelines may say about "dual relationships," when supervisors use the same method as therapists, the actual boundary between therapy and supervision remains inherently ambiguous and a subject of concern (Burns and Holloway 1989). The supervisor can be criticized as being either too therapeutic or not therapeutic enough. More importantly, the inherently ambiguous nature of the supervisor-trainee relationship would eventually pose a host of ethical questions about what constituted proper and improper conduct. For example, a supervisor does not have a clear duty of confidentiality to a supervisee as does a therapist to a patient (Rinas and Clyne-Jackson 1988). Thus, a trainee who confides his or her personal problems to a supervisor in the therapeutic mode may complicate the evaluation process in ways neither of them has anticipated (Whiston and Emerson 1989). The resolution of such ethical problems arising out of dual relationships may have significant legal consequences if there is a noticeably negative impact on the trainee's career. The legal issue would then be whether the trainee was deprived of due process (Cohen and Mariano 1982; Cormier and Bernard 1982).

Video Technology and the Closed-Door Model of Supervision

The norm of weekly face-to-face supervision worked out in psycho-analytic institutes was adopted after World War II. It was used in many psychodynamically oriented training programs in psychiatry, psychology, and social work. The 1958 study by Ekstein and Wallerstein was an important benchmark of that era. Typically, these beginning trainees were not in personal therapy. Their unconscious or even conscious countertransference problems with patients, though frequently mentioned, seldom received systematic attention. This may explain why Ekstein and Wallerstein were proponents of the therapeutic dimension of supervision, although much more sub-tle in their approach than their psychoanalytic predecessors who asked trainees to free-associate. However, given the therapeutic di-mension, there was much discussion about the trainee's transference to the supervisor.

An interesting factual assumption entered the lore of supervision at this time and was later elaborated on (Doehrman 1976; Hora 1957): "It seems to be a well-known phenomenon that therapists often behave in supervision in the same way the patient behaves in therapy" (Moldawsky 1980). The trainee's transference to the super-visor supposedly mirrored, or in some way reflected, his or her rela-tionship to the patient. The intuitive supervisor thus might have access to the deeper and crucial information that was unwittingly reproduced in the supervision session.

The basic issue in any psychotherapy supervision is the kind of information the supervisee brings to the enterprise. Because confidentiality and privacy were sacrosanct values in psychotherapy, the trainee's efforts took place behind closed doors. Furthermore, it was widely assumed by psychoanalytically oriented therapists that the presence of a third-party observer would be a serious impediment to any psychotherapy. Even full disclosure to the patient of the existence of the third-party supervisor was considered detrimental to the treatment by some authorities (DeBell 1963). There were similar objections to recording devices. Of course, if the supervision encounter actually paralleled the trainee's therapeutic encounter with the patient, the crucial information was available. For the many who were unconvinced, the so-called process notes of psychotherapy sessions became the standard medium for supervision (Grinberg 1970).

The trainee would read to the supervisor his or her laborious attempts to write down every significant thing that was said in the session. Process notes might be written during or after sessions (Langs 1980). Because it was difficult for the therapist to talk and to write at the same time, the process notes written during sessions often failed to record what the therapist had said. Process notes written after sessions were subject to other distortions (Schlessinger 1966).

Furthermore, this was the era of training in which the ideal therapist was either the psychoanalyst who offered the patient a neutral screen or the nondirective Rogerian therapist. Many student psychotherapists either followed those ideals in their initial efforts or, if they did not, typically underreported their more voluble interventions. Any trainee could consciously withhold information, and the few trainees who were engaging in inappropriate behavior with their patients could certainly conceal it from their supervisor (Hassenfeld 1987). Empirical research demonstrated that trainee process notes for supervision often left out important themes and provided an inadequate picture of the therapist-patient interaction (Muslin et al. 1967).

The supervisors, who practiced a method of supervision analogous to the dominant Freudian or Rogerian treatment methods, were often neutral and nondirective listeners. Trainees were unlikely to be confronted or to be given negative evaluation feedback (Hassenfeld 1987). Many trainees saw their supervisors as role models and ideal psychotherapists based on how supportively they themselves were treated in supervision (Grinberg 1970). But they had no more opportunity to observe their supervisors as therapists with disturbed and less cooperative patients than the supervisors had to observe the trainees.

Such "closed-door" supervision became the dominant method for teaching psychotherapy and was highly valued by trainees. However, there has never been objective evidence that it was an effective or efficient method for training psychotherapists (Burns and Holloway 1989; Lambert 1980; Robiner and Schofield 1990). Certainly the typically low profile of the therapist trainee, as revealed in closed-door supervision, made it difficult to monitor the particular qualities the trainee brought to the therapeutic exchange. Often, as empirical research demonstrated (Muslin et al. 1967), it was also difficult for the supervisor to assess the patient's clinical condition. When the trainee withheld relevant information (Hassenfeld 1987), it was virtually impossible to identify early signs of the trainee's incompetent or unethical conduct. The pedagogical value of the closed-door approach was harshly criticized by Haley (1977) and by other more active and directive psychotherapists. As it has become clear that the supervisor might be liable for the trainee's failings and for any negative consequences to the patient, the professional adequacy of closed-door supervision confronted a serious challenge on both legal and ethical grounds.

Of course, many training programs in psychotherapy recognized that the beginning psychotherapist needed much more than closed-door supervision. Senior clinicians interviewed patients in conference settings, behind one-way mirrors, and on audiotape; and trainees were expected to do the same (Anderson and Brown 1955). Carl Rogers had already reported his enthusiasm for "Electrically Recorded Interviews" in 1942. Rogers (1957) is also credited with introducing role-playing and simulation techniques. Demonstrations by teachers allowed the student-trainee to be an apprentice who could actually model his or her own approach on that of "human" teachers. It is worth noting that most of the highly respected psychotherapy educators of this era were clinicians who regularly permitted their trainees to observe them in these ways.

This form of teaching psychotherapy by role-modeling was neglected in some training programs. This was particularly so in advanced psychoanalytic training, where the absolute importance of confidentiality and the concern about disrupting the process of free association and transference remained primary considerations. Although psychoanalytic training is more demanding than any other form of psychotherapy, most American psychoanalysts observe only the analytic technique of their own analyst. However valuable that personal experience may be, it provides a limited and very special exposure to psychotherapeutic technique. Standard psychoanalytic supervision and its offshoots have generally continued to rely on process notes, disdaining the technological innovations that would revolutionize the teaching of psychotherapy (Langs 1980).

The use of audiotape and the one-way mirror permitted a more direct, hands-on psychotherapy teaching and supervision. The supervisor using the one-way mirror could observe the trainee and even intervene through live "bug in the ear," telephone, and knock-on-the-door techniques of supervision (Robiner and Schofield 1990).

The advent of videotape is what really transformed psychotherapy supervision. The medium of videotape is quite extraordinary in what it offers to the trainee as well as the supervisor, bringing the entire sphere of nonverbal communication into focus for both in a way audiotape could never do (Ryan and Budner 1970). The ready availability of videotape equipment opened the closed door and permitted significant shifts in supervisory practice focusing on matters that had previously been almost totally overlooked. The video record can provide the kind of information that early psychoanalytic supervision searched for in free associations from the couch. Moreover, the video may reveal even more about the actual human encounter, the nature of the empathic connection, and the unique social reality of the therapist-patient interaction. That interaction is unavailable even in the free associations of one or both of the participants.

The process of psychotherapy supervision now had its own "microscope." Some would say that the supervisee could for the first time obtain objective feedback about his or her conscious and unconscious interaction with the patient and capacity for empathy. The videotape feedback of what went on outside his or her awareness even allowed the trainee to self-supervise. Video was also an invaluable technological breakthrough for the supervision of group and family therapy. Indeed, many of the innovations in supervision came from those quarters, where the limitations of process notes were inescapably obvious (Haley 1977).

Although a videotape can be more revelatory than the trainee might like, it is not as intrusive on the trainee's personal privacy as is the kind of disclosure that occurs with free association or with other methods that encourage self-revelation (Chodoff 1972). The trainee's problems, as a therapist, can certainly be revealed and discussed. But the trainee is not required to assume the patient role and cross the boundary between supervision and personal treatment to present his or her problem. Nor is the trainee required to accept the reductionist premise that transference to the supervisor is somehow crucial evidence about his or her professional capacity to function as a therapist.

The videotape record thus simultaneously brings the trainee's therapeutic persona into objective focus and yet avoids "dual relationships." It also may help to meet legal responsibility by allowing the supervisor to obtain an independent basis for a judgment about the patient's clinical condition (Rinas and Clyne-Jackson 1988). The latter is an important ethical as well as legal consideration. Most commentators now assert that the supervisor's *primary* ethical responsibility is to the patient, and they believe that he or she cannot fulfill that responsibility without ongoing personal clinical knowledge (Cormier et al. 1982).

Because it is such a revelatory documentation of therapy, videotaping presents the greatest possible invasion of the patient's privacy and right to confidentiality. It may also be the most objective evidence for making judgments about the therapist's professional competence. The trainee can use videotapes to seek a second opinion when the supervisor makes a negative evaluation, just as the supervisor might use them to validate the negative evaluation.

During the era of closed-door supervision, it was not uncommon for patients to have little or no knowledge of the nature and extent of supervision (Cavenar et al. 1980). Rarely was a patient informed that he or she was to have an inexperienced therapist, or given the opportunity to exercise informed consent about the disclosure of information to the supervisor. The open-door approaches make it difficult if not impossible to ignore or conceal these matters. The use of videotape for supervision and teaching therefore raises all of the ethical and legal questions involved in obtaining informed consent when both patient and therapist have strong vested interests (Cormier et al. 1982). Recent controversies to be discussed demonstrate that these problems have not yet been adequately resolved (Stone 1991).

The Waning of Dynamic Psychotherapies and the Identity Crisis of Supervision

More recently, the humanistic and dynamic approaches to psychotherapy that grew out of psychoanalysis have been criticized and rejected because there has been insufficient scientific evidence of their efficacy (Klerman 1990). There is also growing skepticism about the assumption that one generic kind of psychotherapy is suitable for the treatment of all disorders. Long-term psychotherapy is also in decline, because third-party payment and the economic incentives of managed care discourage it. Generic psychodynamic psychotherapy is being supplanted by a variety of more structured methods in which the therapist follows a fixed protocol (Bridge and Bascue 1990). Specific therapies have been devised for specific symptoms or disorders (Barlow et al. 1989; Elkin et al. 1989; Fairburn et al. 1991). Behavioral, cognitive, or interpersonal therapy and other such approaches can now be taught in a format more like traditional classroom education. These "protocol" approaches emphasize short-term treatment. The old norm of long-term weekly, private, face-to-face supervision of the trainee's work with one patient may no longer be appropriate. Different supervisors have quite varied areas of competence applicable to different kinds of patients, and they are warned on legal and ethical grounds not to supervise beyond their area of competence (Cormier and Bernard 1982). Furthermore, the guild interests of the various mental health professions have led them to emphasize in their ethical codes that they can only be supervised by members of their own professional guild. Although some training programs adhere to long-term generic supervision as an organizing structure for the trainee's experience, this will be increasingly difficult to justify in an era of subspecialized approaches.

For all of these reasons, the enterprise of psychotherapy supervision is going through an identity crisis. That crisis is reflected in an uncertainty about human values and belief systems, as the supervisor is repeatedly reminded in the literature that it is "unethical to impose one's belief system on the trainee" (cited in Cormier et al. 1982; Kurpius et al. 1991). No wonder that there is a proliferation of "subspecialization" even within specialities. Thus, we have an increasing variety of subspecialized supervisors for subspecializing trainees using different methods and exercising various belief systems.

From the legal and ethical perspective, the supervision of subspecialized paraprofessionals and nonprofessionals is of particular interest (Simon 1991). The supervisor who is a licensed professional is more likely to be seen as legally responsible for their negligence and a better target for a lawsuit, because in such a case, the professional and not the supervisees usually has a "deep pocket" in the form of malpractice insurance.

Many paraprofessional and nonprofessional psychotherapists are drawn from self-help groups. The major qualification of these psychotherapists is that they have gone through the human ordeal that confronts the person they are trying to help. Typically, they have no academic training. Some of them are drawn from 12-step programs, which have their own explicit therapeutic protocol. Other self-help groups, such as Battered Women, have a political and ideological agenda as part of their belief system. They refuse to define their efforts as therapy if doing so means the victim has a mental disorder. The psychotherapy supervisor, who is bound by his or her ethics not to impose a personal belief system, seems totally anomalous instructing those who believe in these politicized self-help orientations. It is not at all clear what the legal and ethical obligations of the specialized professional supervisor should be when he or she assumes responsibility in a collaborative effort with these nonprofessionals, as increasingly happens in community-based settings.

If the lines of legal responsibility are murky, the economic incentives in malpractice litigation are quite clear. The lawyer who sues will target the "deep pocket," and in this context, that puts the insured mental health professional on the line. Some experts have particularly warned professional psychotherapy supervisors against supervising nonprofessionals and practitioners from other professions, and about the legal risks of taking responsibility in clinical settings where a supervisor has no real opportunity to monitor patients (Simon 1991). Although it is difficult to find reported cases (Appelbaum 1991), such warnings are based on the concern that the psychotherapy supervisor will somehow be found either liable for negligent supervision or vicariously liable for the negligence of those he or she supervises.

Legal Aspects of Supervision

Psychotherapy supervisors may fill a variety of clinical and administrative roles. Presumably, however, their primary educational function is to meet periodically with trainees to discuss the ongoing psychotherapy of one or more patients. None of the few reported cases on the liability of psychotherapy supervisors is based on a claim of negligence regarding that primary educational function.

For example, *Cohen v. State of New York* (382 NYS 2d 128 [1976]) is frequently cited as relevant for psychotherapy supervisors. It is an interesting if somewhat antiquated case. Cohen, a third-year medical student, had been hospitalized in the Downstate Medical Center's psychiatric facility. The day he was released he committed suicide, and his wife subsequently brought suit. The psychiatric ward on which he had been treated was organized around the concept of a therapeutic community and used a team approach involving professionals and nonprofessionals. Authority was delegated by design to nurses and trained attendants. The patients were discussed at team meetings three times a week. The court, instructed by expert witnesses, was skeptical about the adequacy of this whole approach for a suicidal patient like Cohen, and faulted the hospital's policies that did not require "direct management of a patient's treatment by a legally qualified psychiatrist." The actual decision to discharge Cohen was made by a first-year psychiatric resident whom the court concluded was not a qualified psychiatrist. The attending physician, who was a qualified psychiatrist, was criticized by the court for not properly supervising the resident's decision.

The opinion does not even suggest that the attending physician was providing psychotherapy supervision to the resident. The court faulted her for not having made her own evaluation of the patient's suicidal tendencies, and for not "actively supervising the care of the decedent." The court, however, made it clear that the negligence of the attending physician (who conceded that the discharge decision was a mistake) was due to the hospital's misguided policies.

The experts for the decedent had convinced the court that for an acutely suicidal patient like the decedent, reliance on the therapeutic community approach was inappropriate and led to negligent decisions. *Cohen v. State of New York* is one of a number of interesting malpractice decisions in which the plaintiff's experts are in effect repudiating not just the practice of one professional colleague but rather the entire professional approach (Stone 1990). Still, the case demonstrates how courts look at the "chain of command" to locate legal responsibility.

Consider two other frequently cited supervision cases from this perspective. Both occurred in the provision of therapy services by federal employees. Typically, in such lawsuits brought under the Federal Torts Claim Act, the federal government and not the particular negligent employee will be responsible for the monetary damages. Both cases involved therapists who had sexual relations with patients they were counseling. In both cases, the therapist's immediate superior learned of the improper behavior through a complaint. Neither of the superiors, who had supervisory authority, intervened responsibly. Again, there was no suggestion that either supervisor had actually functioned as a psychotherapy supervisor. Their negligence was not that they had provided inadequate psychotherapy supervision. Rather, after a complaint from a third party, they failed to exercise their supervisory authority to investigate and intervene to prevent further damaging involvement. The legal theory in both these cases was that the supervisors were themselves negligent.

However, in the second case, *Simmons v. United States* (805 F2d 1363 [9th Cir. 1986]), the court accepted a second theory of negligence based on vicarious liability. Under certain circumstances the supervisor will be responsible for the negligence of a supervisee even when the supervisor has been faultless. The doctrine of respondeat superior holds the employer responsible for the tortious actions of an employee if they arise in "the scope of employment." Under respondeat superior, a supervisor who is in a position of authority or responsibility may be "responsible for the acts of his or her trainees or assistants" (Austin et al. 1990).

Although the supervisor is not, strictly speaking, the "employer" of the person being supervised, he or she may be held liable for negligence of subordinates under the "borrowed servant" doctrine, if the supervisor is serving in the capacity of "master" (Simon and Sadoff 1992). For example, in the hospital setting, the treating psychiatrist is generally supported by residents, interns, nurses, technicians, and others. Rarely are these support staff formal employees of the treating psychiatrist. Nevertheless, vicarious liability may be imposed on the supervising psychiatrist if 1) the subordinate assisting the psychiatrist was negligent, 2) the psychiatrist possessed the requisite degree of control, and 3) the subordinate was acting within the scope of his or her role as assistant (Simon and Sadoff 1992).

In *Simmons v. United States,* the court held the government liable under both respondeat superior and supervisory negligence theories. According to the court, although the counselor was not authorized to become sexually involved with his clients, the contact occurred in conjunction with his legitimate counseling activities and thus perhaps within the scope of his employment. Courts have obviously struggled over the fairness of respondeat superior liability in the face of such patently improper sexual behavior (see, e.g., *Marston v. Minneapolis Clinic of Psychiatry,* 329 N.W.2d 306 [Minn. 1982]). The law on "scope of employment" varies from state to state (Kapp 1984); in *Simmons,* the court decided the matter would properly go to the jury.

The *Tarasoff* case (*Tarasoff v. Regents of the University of California,* 1974), involving a psychotherapist's failure to warn a third party about a dangerous patient, has also been discussed in the psychotherapy supervision literature. One frequently cited report shows that the supervisor's failure to personally examine the patient was a crucial legal consideration (Slovenko 1980). However, the "supervisor" was the administrative head of the clinic, not a psychotherapy supervisor. As these and other cases would demonstrate, the legal risks accrue to those who have supervisory *authority* and *responsibility* and not to the educational enterprise of psychotherapy supervision.

These cases are certainly relevant to psychotherapy supervisors who have administrative control over trainees and have clinical responsibility for patients. They would be functioning in the more complex paradigm having taken on administrative and bureaucratic obligations. At one time—and it is still the case in some programs—the psychotherapy supervisor functioned as an educational *consultant* to the trainee. The consultant was outside the administrative chain of command and had no direct clinical responsibility, and the trainee was not required to comply with the consultant's advice. Supervision was primarily an opportunity for the supervisee to learn about psychotherapy, rather than an opportunity for the patient to have his or her treatment monitored by a more experienced person. Under this simple paradigm, according to Appelbaum and Gutheil (1991), the psychotherapy supervisor as consultant was less likely to be found legally liable for the negligence of his or her trainees.

However, as was already noted, the growing consensus among those who make guild pronouncements about ethics is that the psychotherapy supervisor's primary responsibility is to the patient. This seems to have undermined the consultant/supervisor distinction as it was originally delineated (Appelbaum and Gutheil 1991). A group of psychologists observed, "the legal and ethical responsibility is the same whether the supervisor is a consultant . . . " (Harrar et al. 1990). We get the impression that the guild's ethical standards were ratcheted up because of the dire warnings about the possible legal liabilities. Ironically, the raised ethical standard makes the finding of legal liability more likely (Austin et al. 1990; Harrar et al. 1990; Tanenbaum and Berman 1990).

Standard of Care for Psychotherapy Supervisors

The supervisor who functions in the complex paradigm is more likely to be vicariously liable in respondeat superior and has a higher standard of care to meet as a supervisor. The professional standard of care for psychotherapy supervisors will ordinarily be determined by the expert testimony of peers. However, the professional standard seems to flow from the aforementioned ethical responsibility to the patient. That ethical responsibility suggests a clinical standard for supervisors of *direct* personal observation of the patient. Further, a paradigm of supervision based on primary responsibility to the patient would be geared to the clinical needs of the patient and not to the orientation, substance, and curricular educational arrangements of the training program. The supervisor would have to be readily available and prepared to intervene clinically and meet directly with the patient. Such clinical responsibility would also require ongoing documentation, and the psychotherapy supervisor who has no written records of his or her efforts will be at a disadvantage in the court. Furthermore, ongoing written records will be necessary to document any negative evaluation of the trainee to guarantee due process. All of the above measures, driven by the concern about legal obligations, have been recommended in the literature on psychotherapy supervision (Austin et al. 1990; Harrar et al. 1990). That literature presumably is at least relevant, if it does not in fact establish the standard of care.

The standard that emerges from the literature on the legal and ethical aspects of psychotherapy supervision would be an unrealistic burden in a busy clinic with trainees who are seeing many patients. On the other hand, if guild ethics proclaim a primary responsibility to the patient, the practices of the past will need to be reconsidered. Gutheil (1992) has recommended that all psychotherapy supervisors should in fact reconsider the extent of their clinical responsibilities and examine the specific terms of their professional duties in any institutional affiliation. The fact that the supervisor is donating his or her services is not decisive in these matters.

Various authors have described specific dos and don'ts for supervisors. The following is slightly modified version of the best available list (Austin et al. 1990).

1. Know the supervisee's competence and your own. Question your own competence and consult.

2. Evaluate *all* cases and document the evaluation and your supervision.
3. Use live or videotape supervision or see the patient periodically.
4. Supervise all major decisions by the supervisee, and make sure that the supervisee keeps records.
5. Provide periodic written evaluations to the trainee. Give negative evaluation when indicated.
6. Know the legal rules about supervision. Some states have laws and regulations in connection with licensing. Also, know the obligations, expectations, and so on of institutions where supervision is based.
7. Have a clear understanding with the supervisee of mutual goals and expectations. Arrange for emergency and out-of-town coverage.
8. Make sure that you have adequate malpractice and liability coverage.

Of course, the supervisor who is confident that his or her role is only that of a consultant would be less concerned by these matters. Furthermore, what have been described are the legal possibilities, not the real world probabilities.

Hospitals, clinics, and other organized providers can be liable as corporate entities for the negligence of their employees in a manner similar to the vicarious liability already discussed. They can also be found directly liable for negligence in the hiring or privileging of staff and negligence in their supervision (Donaldson 1986). The hospital must properly investigate the credentials of trainees and see that they are properly supervised. When psychotherapy trainees are involved, the corporate entity can only fulfill its obligations with the assistance of the psychotherapy supervisor. The supervisor should know the credentials of the supervisee before accepting him or her for supervision.

Literature on the Ethics of the Psychotherapy Supervision

Most of the recent writing on the ethical implications of psychotherapy supervision is found in the guild literature of mental health professionals who are not physicians. Much of it deals with responsibility to the patient and the qualifications of the supervisor. There is now a considerable literature on qualification standards and on the training of supervisors in multiple techniques. Experienced supervisors who are able to maintain an open mind may find that these multiple techniques will enrich their supervisory repertoire.

The major theme in this literature on ethics, as already indicated, deals with "dual relations" and the supervisor's potential misuse of power, with a particular concern about sexual exploitation. Other themes include ethical responsibility to the patient (which has been adequately considered here), and the patient's informed consent to supervision, confidentiality, and marketplace issues. These latter issues are briefly addressed.

Concerns about privacy, confidentiality, and informed consent around psychotherapy supervision are relatively new. Only a decade ago, there were responsible people who were opposed to either revealing the fact of supervision or the identity of the supervisor. Most of this opposition came from psychoanalysts concerned about the transference (DeBell 1963). Whether or not those concerns were valid, the issue of informed consent has taken on such force as an ethical and legal matter that those objections now carry little weight.

There is reason for legal if not ethical concern if the supervisor does not inform the patient of the trainee's status, or see to it that the trainee does (Annas 1980). Patients who object to videotaping or to other procedures necessary for proper supervision should be assisted in finding treatment elsewhere. The use of videotapes for teaching purposes should only be done with the express written consent of the patient (Appelbaum and Gutheil 1991; Stone 1991).

There are a number of marketplace issues relevant to psychotherapy supervisors that can be mentioned only briefly here. It is now considered fraudulent for supervisors to sign insurance forms as though they had provided the service themselves (Kovacs 1987). Psychologists have suggested that it may be appropriate to "cosign the form as supervisor" (Austin et al. 1990). However, any efforts to deceive the third-party payer or other fiscal intermediaries are illegal if not unethical.

Psychotherapy supervisors, like psychotherapists, will have

difficulty dealing with the constraints of managed care. The psychotherapist's and the supervisor's legal and ethical responsibilities do not terminate because the patient can no longer pay the bill.

Dual Relationships

Although psychodynamic therapy is much criticized, psychoanalytic concepts still seem to inform the discussion of dual relationships and ethical transgressions by supervisors. The supervisor is typically said to exploit the transference when he or she engages in a sexual relationship with the trainee (American Psychiatric Association [APA] Ethics Committee 1986; Pope et al. 1990; Upchurch 1985). Supervision is seen as analogous to a parent-child relationship. Alternatively, the concept of transference is replaced by more general terms such as power and dependency, which give a slightly different tone to the discussion.

Here it is sufficient to emphasize that where supervision involves therapeutic parameters, it is reasonable to conclude that transference is evoked (Pope et al. 1990). If the concept of transference applies, then it follows that the supervisor, like the therapist, has a fiduciary obligation to abstain from any personal or sexual relationship, even if the trainee knowingly and voluntarily makes the overtures.

Ethics and the Fiduciary Obligation

Each of the mental health professions has its own principles of ethics (e.g., the National Association of Social Workers, the American Association for Marriage and Family Therapy, the American Psychiatric Association, and the American Psychological Association). Supervisors must also be in compliance with any statutory or regulatory standards that are applicable if they are licensed practitioners. However, just as there is no single code of ethics for psychotherapists, there is none for psychotherapy supervisors.

Nonetheless, many problems in professional ethics, including dual relationships, involve conflicts of interest. A professional with a fiduciary obligation must avoid even the appearance of a conflict of interest with the beneficiary. For example, a financial fiduciary cannot borrow money from a beneficiary even if he or she pays a fair interest rate and faithfully repays the principal. Applying the fiduciary standard to psychotherapists, it is generally accepted that the psychotherapist must avoid using the patient to gratify his or her own needs. The first major malpractice case involving sexual exploitation of a patient clearly recognized that issue (*Roy v. Hartogs,* 366 N.Y.S. 297, 300–301 [1975]). The court, in analyzing whether the psychiatrist should be found guilty of malpractice for having sex with his patient, analogized the relationship to the fiduciary/beneficiary relationship, a higher standard than that applicable to ordinary professional relationships. This fiduciary conception of the psychotherapist's obligation has dominated much of the thinking on this and related ethical questions.

Recent commentary concludes that this standard should apply equally to sexual relationships between supervisor and trainee (Austin et al. 1990; Gutheil 1992). There seems to have been no such standard at work in the past. For example, a 1986 survey of female members of APA Division 12 (Clinical Psychology) found that 17% of all respondents (as graduate students) had been sexually involved with their psychology educators. More than 25% of those educators were acting as clinical supervisors (Harrar et al. 1990). A survey of PGY 4 psychiatric residents revealed that 4.5% of those responding to a survey had been sexually involved with "psychiatric educators." Although the numbers were small, a significant percentage of the educators were supervisors. Some of the psychiatric residents had married their supervisors, but the authors noted that over time, many of the others had come to feel they had been exploited. They urged an ethical prohibition regardless of consent.

Concern about dual relationships in ethical guidelines has gone far beyond mixing supervision and intimate sexual relationships. As was previously discussed, there is a conflict between the role of supervisor and therapist. If in the role of therapist the supervisor encourages the student to reveal a problem of substance abuse, or a variety of other significant symptoms of mental disorder, then the supervisor may find him- or herself in a serious professional and ethical dilemma in evaluating the trainee. Furthermore, the lack of timely negative feedback, which may be the inevitable result of a supportive therapeutic attitude, is reported as the basis of many ethical complaints brought against supervisors. However, based on this discussion of methods of supervision, it seems impossible to draw a clear line. Supervisors should be aware of the problem, but the guilds push too far if they prohibit any crossing of the line, and thus discourage the kind of supportive, positive relationships in which all learning flourishes.

Guild ethicists have also been concerned about the dual relationship of teacher and therapist. Yet in a survey of educators engaged in teaching counseling to students, 72% of faculty members reported having explicitly provided simultaneous personal counseling to their own students (Whiston and Emerson 1989). It has certainly been a common practice for students, trainees, and practitioners to seek out recent teachers and supervisors as psychotherapists for themselves or their family members. There are also many anecdotal accounts of close friendships, joint authorship, and successful research carried out by supervisors and their trainees. All of this is brought into question by a rigid application of the ban on dual relationships.

It is worth reemphasizing that a strict construction of the fiduciary standard applied to dual relationships must reject as irrelevant the positive consequences of a breach (e.g., the success of these dual relationships). Just as it would be wrong for a fiduciary to invest the beneficiary's money in a deal that makes them both a fortune, it would be wrong by such a standard to involve a trainee in a professional endeavor that produces a marvelous professional collaboration. Beyond sexual exploitation and other instances of gross misuse of authority, the ban on dual relationships seems absurd to many commentators (Ryder and Hepworth 1990).

Everywhere in graduate education, there is an effort to encourage in mentoring programs the very kind of dual relationships that have become suspect when they occur between supervisors and trainees. Consider this description of mentoring: "The relationship of mentor to mentee combines elements of role modeling, teaching, support and counseling, and friendship" (Psychiatric News 1992). The lack of such a dual relationship is thought to have been particularly harmful to women and minorities in the professions.

The contrast between ethical prohibitions against dual relationships for supervisors and the prescription of them for mentors demands an explanation. One crucial issue, as has been noted, is transference. Many would argue that transference is present in all psychotherapy supervision contexts, and certainly between mentors and mentees. However, whether or not transference occurs, the mental health professions are increasingly vehement in condemning sex between supervisor and trainee. Sexual exploitation is a matter of legal as well as ethical concern throughout our society. The supervisor who makes sexual overtures to a trainee also risks legal charges of sexual harassment.

The Equal Employment Opportunity Commission's definition of sexual harassment has been adopted by many private employers and universities. It defines sexual harassment as follows:

> [Un]welcome sexual advances, requests for sexual favors, and other verbal or physical conduct of a sexual nature . . . when any one of three criteria is met: 1) submission to such conduct is made either explicitly or implicitly a term or condition of an individual's employment, 2) submission to or rejection of such conduct by an individual is used as the basis for employment decisions affecting such individual, or 3) such conduct has the purpose or effect of unreasonably interfering with an individual's work performance or creating an intimidating, hostile, or offensive working environment.

A controversial aspect of the definition is the word "unwelcome," which was presumably intended to indicate that sex in the workplace, if consensual or "welcome," was not prohibited. However, if consensual sex is the basis of career advancement in psychotherapy training, then it certainly is ethically dubious even if legally acceptable. Legal critics have in fact attacked the use of the term "unwelcome," and consider it legally unacceptable on the grounds that it shifts the inquiry to the subjective question of what the employee welcomed, rather than to the objective question of whether the employer made sexual demands on a quid pro quo basis for career advancement (Estrich 1991).

Even those who do not have absolute objections to sexual involve-ments are nonetheless concerned that the supervisor might be biased in his or her present or subsequent evaluations of the trainee who does or does not consent. Furthermore, other trainees who are aware of such a relationship may believe that the resulting biased evalua-tions make the whole system of evaluation unfair. At a minimum, it would seem ethically appropriate to require the supervisor to termi-nate supervision and all other academic or administrative authority before initiating any sexual overture to any trainee. There has re-cently been a great deal of criticism of sexual or romantic relation-ships between therapists and patients after termination of therapy. It is not clear whether similar objections apply to supervisors and their trainees.

Critics of the rigid rule against dual relationships have emphasized that, unlike therapy, the goal of supervision is to help the trainee to become a colleague (Ryder and Hepworth 1990). A rigid application of the fiduciary rule against dual relationships in matters other than sex is difficult to defend, and even the most rigid ethicists seem to recognize that reality (Harrar et al. 1990). The juxtaposition of the enthusiasm for mentoring and the antagonism against dual relation-ships may temper our judgment about both.

Authors who write about the legal and ethical aspects of profes-sional practice are like bird-watchers, eager to spot every rara avis and add it to their lists. Although the rare species exist, the ordinary practitioner is unlikely to encounter them. The legal risks of psycho-therapy supervision can easily be exaggerated, because given the possibility of vicarious liability, it seems anything can happen. How-ever, the probable risks are certainly much lower. Such risks vary drastically from state to state, and most psychotherapy supervisors are unlikely ever to be sued. The range of measures necessary to avoid the possible liability risks are time consuming and might lead supervisors to radically alter their practices. Although some of these measures have pedagogical value, others do not.

Many training programs that now delegate clinical responsibility to trainees may need to reconsider their malpractice coverage and review the malpractice coverage of supervisors. The literature is filled with warnings about assigning difficult patients to trainees. Yet there are some of us whose experience suggests that what young psychotherapists lack in wisdom is more than compensated for by the other human qualities they bring to psychotherapy. Risk management should not become bureaucratic shackles.

References

American Psychiatric Association Ethics Committee: Sexual involvements between psychiatrists and their students, supervisees, colleagues, co-workers and employees. Washington, DC, American Psychiatric Association, April/May 1986

Anderson RP, Brown OH: Tape recordings and counselor-trainee understandings. Journal of Counseling Psychology 2:189–195, 1955

Annas GJ: The care of private patients in teaching hospitals: legal implications. Bull N Y Acad Med 56:403–411, 1980

Appelbaum PS: General guidelines for psychiatrists who prescribe medication for patients treated by non-medical psychotherapists. Hosp Community Psychiatry 42:281–282, 1991

Appelbaum PS, Gutheil TG: Clinical Handbook of Psychiatry and the Law, 2nd Edition. Baltimore, MD, Williams & Wilkins, 1991

Austin KM, Moline ME, Williams GT (eds): Confronting Malpractice: Legal and Ethical Dilemmas in Psychotherapy. Beverly Hills, CA, Sage, 1990, pp 230–237

Barlow DH, Craske MG, Cerny JA, et al: Behavioral treatment of panic disorder. Behavior Therapy 20:261–282, 1989

Blocher DH: Toward a cognitive developmental approach to counseling supervision. Counseling Psychologist 11(1):27–34, 1983

Bridge P, Bascue LO: Documentation of psychotherapy supervision. Psychotherapy in Private Practice 8(1):79–86, 1990

Burns CI, Holloway EL: Therapy in supervision: an unresolved issue. Clinical Supervisor 7(4):47–59, 1989

Cavenar JR, Jesse O, Rhoads EJ, et al: Ethical and legal aspects of supervision. Bull Menninger Clin 44(1):15–22, 1980

Chodoff P: Supervision of psychotherapy with videotapes: pros and cons. Am J Psychiatry 128:819–823, 1972

Cohen v State of New York, 382 NYS 2d 128, 1976

Cohen RJ, Mariano EM: Legal Guidebook in Mental Health. New York, Free Press, 1982

Cormier LS, Bernard S, Bernard JM: Ethical and legal responsibilities of clinical supervisors. Personnel and Guidance Journal, pp 486–491, April 1982

DeBell DE: A critical digest of the literature on psychoanalytic supervision. American Psychoanalytic Association Journal 11:546–575, 1963

Doehrman MJG: Parallel processes in supervision and psychotherapy. Bull Menninger Clin 40(1):3–104, 1976

Donaldson RG: Hospital's failure to supervise doctor. 12 ALR 4th 57, 1982

Donaldson RG: Liability of hospital or clinic for sexual relationships with patients by staff physicians, psychologists, and other healers. 45 ALR 4th 289, 1986

Ekstein R, Wallerstein RS: The Teaching and Learning of Psychotherapy. New York, International Universities Press, 1958

Elkin E, Shea T, Watkins JT, et al: National Institute of Mental Health Treatment of Depressions Collaborative Research Program: general effectiveness of treatment. Arch Gen Psychiatry 46:971–982, 1989

Estrich S: Sex at work. 43 Stanford Law Review 813, 1991

Fairburn CG, Jones R, Proveler RC, et al: Three psychological treatments for bulimia nervosa: a comparative trial. Arch Gen Psychiatry 48:463–469, 1991

Gartrell N, Herman J, Olartes S, et al: Sexual contact with educators and patients: results of a national survey. Am J Psychiatry 145:690–694, 1988

Grinberg L: The problems of supervision in psychoanalytic education. Int J Psychoanal 51:371–383, 1970

Gutheil T: Clinical Psychiatry News 20(3), March 1992

Haley J: Problem-Solving Therapy: New Strategies for Effective Family Therapy. San Francisco, CA, Jossey-Bass, 1977

Harrar WR, VandeCreek L, Knapp S: Ethical and legal aspects of clinical supervision. Professional Psychology: Research and Practice 21:37–41, 1990

Hassenfeld IN: Ethics and the role of the supervisor of psychotherapy. Journal of Psychiatric Education 11(2):73–77, 1987

Hess AK (ed): Psychotherapy Supervision: Theory, Research and Practice. New York, Wiley, 1980, Chapter 31

Hora T: Contribution to the phenomenology of the supervisory process. Am J Psychother 11:773–796, 1957

Huber CH, Baruth LG: Ethical, Legal and Professional Issues in the Practice of Marriage and Family Therapy. Columbus, OH, Merrill Publishing, 1987

Kapp MB: Supervising professional trainees: legal implications for mental health institutions and practitioners. Hosp Community Psychiatry 35:143–147, 1984

Klerman GL: The psychiatric patient's right to effective treatment: implications of *Osheroff v. Chestnut Lodge*. Am J Psychiatry 147:409–418, 1990

Kovacs AL: Insurance billing: the growing risk of lawsuits against psychologists. Independent Practitioner 7:21–24, 1987

Kurpius D, Gibson G, Lewis J, et al: Ethical issues in supervising counseling practitioners. Counselor Education and Supervision 31(1):48–57, 1991

Lambert MJ: Psychotherapy Supervision: Theory, Research and Practice. Edited by Hess AK. New York, Wiley, 1980

Langs RJ: in Psychotherapy Supervision: Theory, Research and Practice. Edited by Hess AK. New York, Wiley, 1980

Loganbill C, Hardy E, Delworth U: Supervision: a conceptual model. Counseling Psychologist 10(1):3–42, 1982

Marston v Minneapolis Clinic of Psychiatry, 329 NW 2d 306, Minn 1982

Minnes PM: Ethical issues in supervision. Canadian Psychology 28(3):285–290, 1987

Moldawsky S: Psychoanalytic psychotherapy supervision, in Psychotherapy Supervision: Theory, Research and Practice. Edited by Hess AK. New York, Wiley, 1980

Muslin HL, Burstein AG, Gedo JE, et al: Research on the supervisory process, I: supervisor's appraisal of the interview data. Arch Gen Psychiatry 16:427–431, 1967

Nemiah JC: Supervision: teaching or psychotherapy? Canada's Mental Health Supplement 66:3–6, 1971

Perkes GT: Medical malpractice—ostensible agency and corporate negligence—hospital liability may be based on either doctrine of ostensible agency or doctrine of corporate negligence. St Mary's Law Journal 17:551–578, 1986

Pope KS, Schover LR, Levenson H: Sexual behavior between clinical supervisors and trainees: implication for professional standards. Professional Psychology 157–162, February 1990

Psychiatric News, July 3, 1992, p 16

Rinas J, Clyne-Jackson S: Professional Conduct and Legal Concerns in Mental Health Practice. Norwalk, CT, Appleton & Lange, 1988

Robiner WN, Schofield W: References on supervision in clinical and counseling psychology. Professional Psychology: Research and Practice 21(4):297–312, 1990

Robiner WN, Fuhrman MJ, Bobbit BL: Supervision in the practice of psychology: toward the development of a supervisory instrument. Psychotherapy in Private Practice 8:87–98, 1990

Rogers CR: The use of electrically recorded interviews in improving psychotherapeutic techniques. Am J Orthopsychiatry 12:429–443, 1942

Rogers CR: Training individuals to engage in the therapeutic process, in Psychology and Mental Health. Edited by Strother CR. Washington, DC, American Psychological Association, 1957, pp 76–92

Rogers CR: Non-directive psychotherapy, in Psychotherapy Supervision: Theory, Research and Practice. Edited by Hess AK. New York, Wiley, 1980

Roy v Hartogs, 366 N.Y.S. 297, 300–301, 1975

Ryan JH, Budner S: Impact of television: an evaluation of the use of videotapes in psychiatric training. Am J Psychiatry 126:1397–1403, 1970

Ryder R, Hepworth J: AAMFT ethical code: "dual relationships." Journal of Marital and Family Therapy 16(2):127–132, 1990

Schlessinger N: Supervision of psychotherapy—a critical review of the literature. Arch Gen Psychiatry 15:129–134, 1966

Simmons v United States, 805 F2d 1363, 9th Cir. 1986

Simon RI (ed): Review of Clinical Psychiatry and the Law, Vol 2. Washington, DC, American Psychiatric Press, 1991

Simon RI, Sadoff RL: Psychiatric Malpractice: Cases and Comments for Clinicians. Washington, DC, American Psychiatric Press, 1992, pp 33–51

Slovenko R: Psychotherapy Supervision: Theory, Research and Practice. Edited by Hess AK. New York, Wiley, 1980

Stone AA: Law, science, and psychiatric malpractice: a response to Klerman's indictment of psychoanalytic psychiatry. Am J Psychiatry 147:419–427, 1990

Stone AA: Confidentiality in psychotherapy—the case of Anne Sexton. N Engl J Med 325(20):1450, 1991

Tanenbaum RL, Berman MA: Ethical and legal issues in psychotherapy supervision. Psychotherapy in Private Practice 8(1):65–77, 1990

Tarasoff v Regents of the University of California, 118 Cal Rptr 129, 529 P2d 553, 1974

Upchurch DW: Professional issues: ethical standards and the supervisory process. Counselor Education and Supervision 25(2):90–98, 1985

Van Hoose WH, Kottler JA: Ethical and Legal Issues in Counselling and Psychotherapy, 2nd Edition. San Francisco, CA, Jossey-Bass, 1985

Whiston SC, Emerson S: Ethical implications for supervisors in counseling of trainees. Counselor Education and Supervision 28:318–325, 1989

Chapter 3

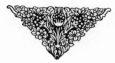

Gender Issues in Supervision

Carol C. Nadelson, M.D.,
Catherine Belitsky, M.D., F.R.C.P.C.,
Mary V. Seeman, M.D., F.R.C.P.C., and
Keith Ablow, M.D.

Our focus in this chapter is on the influence of gender on the supervisory process. We consider the interactions of supervisors, supervisees, and patients. Although the specific literature on this topic is sparse, the framework in which to understand this process can benefit from interactional concepts derived from sociology.

The Impact of Gender on Communication

Deaux and Major (1987) provide a useful theoretical framework. They suggest that each of the two individuals in a relationship presents him- or herself using language and behavior that convey a pre-existing self-ascribed gender role and, in addition, conform to the perceived expectations of the other. Thus, the manifestations of gender identity shift depending on the two persons involved and, to a certain extent, on context. In clinical work, this shift may be subtle, but it can lead to behavior that compromises both the learning process and patient care. For example, a supervisor may hold expectations that supervisees are heterosexual or that they do not uphold radical feminist views. Such preconceived ideas can undermine a preexisting gender role in the supervisee and lead away from honest interchange into pretense and inauthenticity.

▼ Pretending to Be What One Is Expected to Be

A trainee who was in a long-term lesbian relationship was being supervised by a male supervisor who assumed that she was heterosexual. When the trainee presented a therapy case involving a homosexual male couple, the supervisor suggested that the relationship itself reflected pathology and made gratuitous remarks intended to be humorous. The trainee considered complaining to the training director. Not wanting to risk the possibility that he might share her supervisor's perspective, however, she decided to be careful to avoid any reference to her own personal life or her feelings about sexual issues in her patients. She tailored her subsequent supervisory sessions and carefully selected both her cases for presentation and the vocabulary she used in reporting them. In other words, she presented herself more or less as she perceived her supervisor expected her to be in the context of their supervisory hour.

The Deaux and Major (1987) model emphasizes context. In situations like supervision in which there is a teaching relationship, where the supervisee seeks to learn from the more experienced supervisor, he or she is more likely to present in ways designed to please the supervisor. For example, a woman trainee may unconsciously exaggerate stereotypical female traits that are culturally accepted—traits she has learned from experience are a means of attracting positive attention and assistance. This can blur the supervisory boundaries and limit the free flow of information.

Another instance of the information screening effect of gender stereotypes can be seen in the following example.

▼ Avoiding Anticipated Gender Bias

A male patient was in therapy because of the legal repercussions of having exposed himself to women passersby on a beach. He saw his behavior as no different from that of women who wear short skirts or tight sweaters. Showing his penis to women, he reasoned, should arouse them in the same way that a women's breasts or bare legs might arouse men.

The female therapist was reluctant to discuss this with her male supervisor because she thought that this material might lead to a discussion of why women wore "seductive" clothes. She was especially sensitive about the issue, because her supervisor had, on many occasions, made her uncomfortable by remarking on what she herself wore.

Gender, Clinical Work, and Learning

In supervision, there are three individuals involved: the patient, the trainee, and the supervisor. Scher (1981) critically examined the various combinations of gender roles that this situation creates. Changing perspectives on the roles and aspirations of women and men serve as possible areas of conflict at the different levels of the triad. Such conflict can cloud objectivity in diagnosis and treatment approach, in evaluations, and in disclosure of relevant clinical material (Boggiano and Barrett 1991; Loring and Powell 1988; Munson 1987; Nelson 1991; Nieva and Gutek 1980).

Misinterpretation of meaning or the confusion of roles is another area where gender values may affect supervision, as seen in the following instance.

▼ Supervisor-Trainee Boundaries

A male supervisor took a female trainee to lunch. Noticing that the supervisor was wearing a wrinkled shirt, she made a good-natured remark about his appearance. He responded by telling her that his wife was sick and unavailable to him. The trainee listened sympathetically and encouraged him to speak more about his dissatisfaction with his wife. He then confided that the two of them had been distant for a long time prior to her illness. "That sounds perfectly horrible," the trainee offered. "You deserve better."

The supervisor misinterpreted her apparent interest and inquired as to whether the two might talk at greater length over dinner. The supervisee was uncomfortable. But because she was feeling that her own comments, even though misinterpreted, began the interaction, she accepted the invitation. She also believed that she could not refuse because, if she did, her evaluation might suffer and this could affect her future career. Thus, she not only felt coerced into a social relationship that she did not want, but she did not get the supervision she needed.

Subsequently, when this supervisee, feeling distressed about the interaction, reported the incident to a female supervisor, the supervisor suggested that perhaps she had been more seductive in her behavior than she realized and that she was overreacting to the incident. This interpretation added to the supervisee's distress and was not useful to her when she needed help in understanding how boundary violations arise.

In situations like this, it is the responsibility of the supervisor to maintain these boundaries and to provide an environment that is conducive to learning. It is important that both trainees and staff understand this.

Other aspects of supervision that are affected by gender and gender roles can be seen in some same-sex supervisory pairs. Competitive male-male behavior can result in a male trainee finding himself acting in stereotypically exaggerated dominant, assertive, and uncompromising ways, thus impeding the supervisory dialogue.

▼ Supervisor-Trainee Competitiveness

A male trainee seemed to make it a point of honor never to ask for guidance or assistance from his supervisor. When such guidance was offered, he reacted defensively and with irritation.

Although the supervisor was very concerned about some of the clinical decisions made by the trainee, he was careful not to appear judgmental. The supervisor approached the problem not by challenging the trainee's decisions but by creating an atmosphere that was more congenial to the sharing of ideas than to competing. "You're experienced at this work now," he said to the trainee on one occasion. "What would have been another way for you to respond to that patient?" This empathic and supportive approach seemed to work and allowed the supervisee to gradually abandon his competitive stance.

Although women supervisors are now commonplace, some men continue to be uncomfortable "subordinating" themselves to a woman. Several authors address avoidance of certain issues in the male trainee/female supervisor/female patient triad and warn about potential harmful clinical effects (Alonso and Rutan 1978; Brodsky 1980; Mendell 1986; Nadelson and Notman 1977; Scher 1981). They also point to the potential for growth in the trainee, and to improved patient outcome when this triad functions optimally. Abramowitz and Abramowitz (1976) address the potential pitfalls in the all-woman triad. Leighton (1991) and Kaplan (1985) identify some difficulties in stereotypical "masculine" supervisory styles. They suggest that women in general may be more intuitive and more conscious of relational issues than men and therefore are to be preferred as supervisors, especially around "female issues" in psychotherapy. Further elucidation of the advantages and disadvantages of gender congruity and incongruity in supervision will clearly be helpful as gender issues are better understood.

Women patients frequently feel that fears of rape, victimization, abortion, and body image distortion are not empathically understood by men and are inadequately responded to. It is possible that a male supervisor would not be as sensitive about the implications of these experiences, especially if his training did not include substantive discussion of these issues. The reverse may hold for male patients. Gender congruence and gender-orientation congruence may prove to be important to clinical outcome.

▼　The Need to Identify With a Supervisor

A trainee who was gay presented a case where his patient, who was also gay, was in the process of "coming out." The supervisor, who was Jewish, equated the process with one he was more familiar with—the denial of Jewishness and the attempt to pass as a Christian in a Christian world. The trainee thought the analogy was imprecise and that the supervisor was imposing his own frame of reference onto an experience that he knew nothing about. The trainee felt misunderstood and asked to be supervised by a gay supervisor.

Advantages to sex incongruence in supervision have also been stressed (Nelson 1991). Essentially, it has been noted that supervision by a member of the opposite sex can identify some sex-based biases that a supervisor of the same sex may miss. Thus, it seems important that supervisees have supervisors of both sexes and from diverse backgrounds whenever possible.

One of the most problematic issues in the supervisory relationship is the possibility—sometimes the fact—of the transformation of this teacher-student partnership into a sexual union. Most writers agree that a power differential exists between trainee and supervisor and that this precludes free consent (Brodsky 1980). A recent survey of Canadian psychiatric residents found that 9.7% of female residents reported incidents of sexual harassment during their training (Carr et al. 1991). Male residents reported no incidents. Of the respondents in this survey (which had a 58.7% response rate), 2.5% reported sexual involvement with a faculty member, although 13.1% reported being propositioned. The involvement was not viewed as negative in the majority of cases; but the eventual outcome, as suggested by Pope and colleagues (1979), may be disrespect for boundaries in therapy situations. Robinson and Reid (1985) and Glaser and Thorpe (1986) also discuss trainee-supervisor sexual involvement and its repercussions.

▼ Consenting Adults

A medical student who was planning a career in psychiatry received a failing grade in an elective. Because she had always been an excellent student, this inconsistency was questioned by her faculty advisor. After a long silence and considerable reluctance to discuss the topic, the student revealed that the course director had made a pass at her. Subsequently, she felt so uncomfortable that she stopped going to the elective, provoking the failing grade. When the course director was confronted, he emphasized that the student was an adult and that the advisor had no jurisdiction in the "business" of two adults.

It is worth noting in the context of this example that the survey by Carr and colleagues (1991) indicated that educator-student boundary violations were not discussed in the vast majority of Canadian post-graduate training programs in psychiatry.

Many legal and ethical issues are raised by gender-related considerations. In an environment of embarrassment or sexual tensions, key issues may be avoided in supervision. These issues may also have legal ramifications.

▼ Sexual Embarrassment

A senior male psychology student, presenting the case of a 39-year-old woman in psychotherapy for a dysphoric disorder, omitted the patient's reproductive history. The supervisor did not ask for it. When the therapy did not progress, therapist and supervisor hypothesized about the reasons. Only much later did they realize that the questions the therapist had not asked out of embarrassment were key to understanding the patient.

Sexual Abuse of Patients

One of the most difficult problems facing clinicians is the knowledge of sexual abuse of patients by colleagues. Trainees are often aware of its occurrence among their peers. Occasionally they hear from patients that sexual involvement occurred in the past, sometimes with a prominent faculty member. Trainees do not know what to do with such information. They may or may not know the legal, ethical, and clinical implications of the behavior. It is important that training programs acknowledge the seriousness of these gender-related issues and stress the potential role of the supervisory process in disseminating and assimilating sensitive and emotionally disturbing ethical imperatives.

Gender in Resident Selection and Evaluation of Supervisors

Among the gender issues that are infrequently considered are the influences of gender on the selection and evaluation of supervisors. In interviewing psychiatric residents from training programs in the

Boston area, one of the authors (K.A.) found that, when given a choice, reputation and perceived power were primary indices by which residents chose supervisors. The degree of prominence or celebrity achieved by senior clinicians consistently emerged as more important to residents than the supervisor's sex, educational background, number of publications, or theoretical orientation. Thus, a female supervisor who was widely considered interesting, insightful, gifted, and dedicated to teaching would more likely be chosen by both male and female trainees over a less well-regarded male supervisor. Residents positively regard high-ranking faculty members; but given supervisors with equal reputations, female residents preferred to have a balance of male and female supervisors, whereas male residents preferred male supervisors.

Among the other issues that emerged from this survey was the observation that residents positively regarded supervisors who were known to have "strong" personalities and to express this in the work setting, whether by eloquently and forcefully voicing their opinions, refining a charismatic professional style, talking openly about compelling outside interests, or otherwise making themselves known as individuals. For a variety of reasons, this style may be more common (and perhaps more tolerated by colleagues) among male faculty members.

Another influence appeared to be sex role definition. Male and female trainees positively regarded same-sex supervisors who displayed more stereotypic gender-specific behaviors, including styles of speech and appearance, in the work environment. Like the presence of a "strong" personality, this seemed to buffer the resident's fear of being homogenized or "desexed" by psychiatric training. Male residents (especially those who were heterosexual) appeared to gravitate toward male supervisors who were physically imposing, who occasionally used crude language, or who were interpersonally aggressive. Male residents used terms like "straight shooter," "regular guy," and "intense" to describe supervisors they considered highly desirable. A female resident, on the other hand, commented that the stylish dress of one of her supervisors had attracted her. She saw this as evidence that the supervisor "still had a sense of herself" and had not been "turned into a man."

Residents of both sexes appeared to reject stereotypically masculine behavior in female supervisors and stereotypically feminine behavior in male supervisors. The few homosexual residents interviewed did not have this bias.

With regard to sexual orientation, heterosexual residents appeared to negatively regard homosexuality in supervisors of either sex. The use of derogatory terms in descriptions of these supervisors was not uncommon. Homosexual residents of both sexes tended to seek out homosexual supervisors of either sex.

Residents generally had negative reactions to male or female faculty members who withheld their time or affect. It did appear, however, that even routine competing demands on a faculty member's time were less easily forgiven by residents in women faculty members, of whom a more nurturing style might be expected, as of women in general.

It appears, then, that maintaining stereotyped gender-specific behaviors in the professional environment may be more prized than ability or supervisory skill. A supervisor cannot easily overcome these biases by virtue of technical competence alone. It also appears that gender issues not only affect selection of supervisors, but they also influence resident evaluation of supervisors. The model described by Deaux and Major (1987) would have predicted these results.

Recommendations

Some recommendations derive from the issues discussed in this chapter. First, supervisors and supervisees need to increase their sensitivity to gender issues. It is the responsibility of the training program to ensure that this occurs. Second, male and female trainees can benefit from being supervised by both male and female supervisors. Training program directors need to be proactive in promoting this value.

Because the trainee begins to master the complexity of the psychotherapeutic endeavor with its challenges and rewards through exposure to supervision, a range of supervisors representing many views needs to be provided. Each of the mental health disciplines in most schools in North America has more than adequate numbers of well-qualified women and men to provide the necessary supervisory balance.

Exposure of trainees to differences in perspective and in emphasis enhances their experience. Despite the increase in complexity and the potential for added confusion, psychotherapy demands continuing reappraisal and reexamination of all aspects of the therapeutic encounter, including gender-related aspects.

As we have emphasized in this chapter, supervision is a larger and more inclusive responsibility than is sometimes acknowledged. The supervisor serves as a role model for therapeutic work with patients and for lifelong self-examination. The perspectives and perceptions of peers and colleagues of both sexes and both sexual orientations would enrich the humanity of psychotherapeutic work and can only improve clinical outcomes.

References

Abramowitz SI, Abramowitz CV: Sex role psychodynamics in psychotherapy supervision. Am J Psychother 30:583–592, 1976

Alonso A, Rutan S: Cross-sex supervision for cross-sex therapy. Am J Psychiatry 135:928–931, 1978

Boggiano AK, Barrett M: Strategies to motivate helpless and mastery-oriented children: the effect of gender-based expectancies. Sex Roles 25:487–510, 1991

Brodsky AM: Sex role issues in the supervision of therapy, in Psychotherapy Supervision: Theory, Research and Practice. Edited by Hess AK. New York, Wiley, 1980

Carr ML, Robinson GE, Stewart DE, et al: A survey of Canadian psychiatric residents regarding resident-educator sexual contact. Am J Psychiatry 148:216–220, 1991

Deaux K, Major B: Putting gender into context: an interactive model of gender-related behavior. Psychol Rev 94:369–389, 1987

Glaser RD, Thorpe JS: Unethical intimacy: a survey of sexual contact and advances between psychology educators and female graduate students. Am Psychol 41:43–51, 1986

Kaplan AG: Female or male therapists for women patients: new formulations. Psychiatry 48:111–121, 1985

Leighton J: Gender stereotyping in supervisory styles. Psychoanal Rev 78:347–363, 1991

Loring M, Powell B: Gender, race, and DSM-III: a study of the objectivity of psychiatric diagnostic behavior. J Health Soc Behav 29:1–22, 1988

Mendell D: Cross-gender supervision of cross-gender therapy: female supervisor, male candidate, female patient. Am J Psychoanal 46:270–275, 1986

Munson CE: Sex roles and power relationships in supervision. Professional Psychology: Research and Practice 18:236–243, 1987

Nadelson C, Notman M: Psychotherapy supervision: the problem of conflicting values. Am J Psychother 31:275–283, 1977

Nelson TS: Gender in family therapy supervision. Contemporary Family Therapy 13:357–369, 1991

Nieva VF, Gutek BA: Sex effects on evaluation. Academy of Management Review 5:267–276, 1980

Pope KS, Levenson H, Schover LR: Sexual intimacy in psychology training: results and implications of a national survey. Am Psychol 34:682–689, 1979

Robinson WL, Reid PT: Sexual intimacies in psychology revisited. Professional Psychology 16:512–520, 1985

Scher M: Gender issues in psychiatric supervision. Compr Psychiatry 22:179–183, 1981

Chapter 4

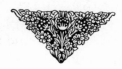

Issues in Psychotherapy Supervision When Participants Are From Different Cultures

Ronald Ruskin, M.D., F.R.C.P.C.

Homo sum; humani nil a me alienum puto.
[I am a man. I count nothing human foreign to me.]

Terence (c. 190–159 B.C.)

Psychotherapy supervision may be defined as an interactive learning process between the psychotherapy supervisor and the supervisee (resident), with the object of study being the supervisee's therapeutic work. This supervisory process frequently takes place in a hospital or a psychotherapy (i.e., psychoanalytic) training program and is therefore influenced by the predominant perspectives and values shaped by the training program. Arlow (1963) has commented on the uniqueness of the supervisory situation in that it comprises the opportunity to observe, "all at the same time, a group of simultaneous interactions; the interac-

I thank Dr. Leo Chagoya and Dr. Marlinda Friere for their assistance in the preparation of this chapter.

tion between patient and therapist (P ↔ T), between therapist and supervisor (T ↔ S), and finally the subtle effect of the organizational relationship to the institute" (p. 577). Ekstein and Wallerstein (1972) have referred to this schema of patient (P), therapist (T), supervisor (S), and administrator (A) as linked in the form of a "clinical rhombus" that reflects the "different functions that the participants carry" (p. 11; see Figure 4–1). This schema, however, is not simply a fixed external structure, but a rather fluid series of internal self and object representations that may shift according to dynamic pressures within each participant. A further determinant (which has rarely been commented on) is that of cultural experience and the extent to which such experience influences each participant in the clinical rhombus, and therefore the efficacy and outcome of the supervisory situation.

Each participant in this external configuration (Figure 4–2) may therefore be experienced in innumerable ways according to both external and internal phenomena that include his or her respective cultural determinants. As Foulks (1980) put it:

> Culture plays a major role in shaping how we think, behave, feel. Culture determines how and by whom children are raised, how they are fed . . . how they acquire roles of behavior, how they are punished, and how they learn about sex, gender roles, and marriage. Culture may affect personal psychology and shape

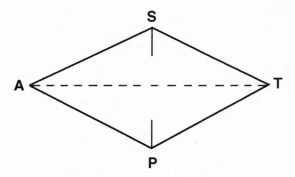

Figure 4–1. The clinical rhombus after Ekstein and Wallerstein (1972). P = patient, T = therapist-supervisee, S = supervisor, A = administrator.

character. Culture provides standards and values according to how one evaluates one's self, one's group, and outsiders. Culture provides guidelines and rules for recognizing and diagnosing emotional illness, for its management, and at times, its treatment. (p. 812)

For the purposes of this chapter, culture is defined from an ethnocultural perspective, including racial, religious, linguistic, and certain other traits held in common (Collins 1984). I examine the uniqueness of psychotherapy supervision when the patient (P), therapist-supervisee (T), and supervisor (S) comes from different ethnocultural backgrounds. It is hypothesized that there is an increased likelihood of supervisory difficulties and unsatisfactory experiences within the supervisory relationship if different participant orientations are not appropriately discussed or worked through. Traditionally, difficulties or impasses within supervision are perceived to arise when external conflicts and anxieties related to transference/countertransference issues cannot be fully explored, empathically felt, and adequately worked through. Cultural issues may

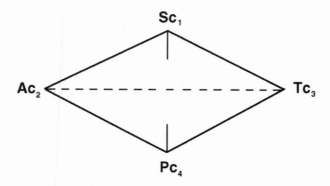

Figure 4–2. The influence of cultural determinants (C), where C may differ in each individual.
P = patient, T = therapist-supervisee, S = supervisor, A = administrator, and C_1, C_2, C_3, and C_4 may represent racial, linguistic, religious, or national factors.

represent another level of discourse that takes its social origins from outside the supervisory relationship. Nonetheless, these issues impinge on the capacity of therapist-supervisee and supervisor to understand and monitor their responses to each other.

Cultural differences may strongly influence, for example, the manner in which a person treats a student or a teacher, and such differences regulate the degree of role responsiveness within an educational institution. Psychodynamic factors interact with cultural determinants, and the capacity of both supervisor and supervisee to attend to such issues may contribute toward responsiveness or nonresponsiveness within the supervisory relationship. Case material is presented here to support the relevance of cultural determinants in psychotherapy supervision.

Patient-Therapist Interaction: Early Psychotherapy Studies

The area of cultural difference is minimally represented in the psychotherapy and supervision literature. Obendorf (1954) drew attention to conditions in mental illness "which require special considerations of race, creed, and color before they can be even gently touched. Special knowledge in two particulars, at least, is necessary for effective treatment—linguistics and an understanding of racial heritages" (p. 754). Obendorf went on to discuss that the possession of intellectual knowledge was a necessary but not sufficient condition for this type of work. The psychiatrist's character and "disposition to convey confidence" to the patient was an essential need. Obendorf advanced the idea that having psychiatrists of various creeds and nationalities would help fulfill this need. As an ideal, any psychiatrist who had undergone psychoanalysis should be free of "blind spots and biases," yet this seemed to be a "practical impossibility." Obendorf offered a reprobation for private therapists (analysts) who were definitely not socially minded. From a therapeutic standpoint, "transference in its positive form is *most likely* to be established and examined (analyzed) between patient and hospital and patient and physician if their psychological biases do not differ too widely" (p. 757, italics added).

Writing from a Kleinian perspective, Jacques (1955) described that one of the primary cohesive elements binding individuals into human institutionalized associations is that of a defense against psychotic anxiety. Defenses against persecutory anxiety—such as splitting into good/bad objects, maintaining the sense of the idealized good object within, and projecting the sense of the bad object outward—may operate at either the level of a cultural group or the individual. Cultural differences may be particularly used by the patient, therapist, or supervisor, to project unacceptable impulses into the other and identify that other individual for the purposes of attack or derision. Schacter and Butts (1968), in contrast to Obendorf, believe that difficulties involved in interracial (therapy) analysis may be no greater than analyses when race is not an issue. However, they suggest that the "confluence of countertransference and stereotypes serves to delay the analysis" (p. 817). Describing interracial analysis, Fischer (1971) states, "racial differences between analyst and analysand involve issues of unconscious meaning at many levels. These issues and meanings must be recognized and utilized, for there are serious hazards in either overestimating or ignoring them" (p. 737).

Cavenar and Spaulding (1978), citing the successful psychotherapeutic treatment of a white male by a black female, believe that interracial therapy can be as productive as any other psychotherapy:

> The same conflicts must be worked through in this kind of interracial therapy—as in any other treatment, the sequence of the unfolding of the conflicts may be altered by racial issues. Differences in race may serve as a scaffold for multiple projections by the patient. Projections pertaining to race must be dealt with early in the treatment by helping the patient to appreciate these are unconscious conflicts. (p. 1086)

Brantley (1983) recommends that the racial issue should not be minimized. Varghese (1983) mentions that "failure to appreciate the impact of racial differences can impede therapeutic progress, while sensitive confrontation may be a valuable tool in the recognition and communication of emotionally charged feelings in therapy" (p. 329). Varghese also found evidence in reviewing his process notes of his own failure to confront early references to racial difference and bring them to the attention of himself and his supervisor. He added:

> Often the trainee's failure to bring up racial issues in supervision is matched by the *supervisor's unwillingness* to mention it. Discussion of racial differences in supervisory sessions will serve not only to make the trainee therapists aware of the impact of their persons on their patients but also encourage self-understanding and growth as trainees develop identities as psychotherapists. (Varghese 1983, p. 332, italics added)

Holmes (1992) reiterated that a therapist may not fully interpret intrapsychic conflicts in the "face of racial explanations offered by patients-[*if they*] induce white therapist guilt, black therapist overidentification with the downtrodden (a particular form of countertransference problem) and ward off aggression in that therapist." (p. 1; italics added)

The general consensus of these authors is that cultural determinants (specifically, interracial factors) are amenable to psychotherapy, provided the therapist is able to effectively recognize bias and sensitively deal with transference/countertransference issues. In addition, Myers (1988) importantly points out that the patient or supervisee may use racial or cultural differences between the two parties as a resistance to the awareness of underlying transference/countertransference effects or latent psychodynamic content. On another level, the psychotherapy supervisor's recognition that cultural factors play a significant role in therapy and the supervisory process can enhance his or her capacity to facilitate such communications. Obendorf's (1954) comments on the special requirements of the psychiatrist—linguistics and an understanding of racial heritages—as well as a "disposition to convey confidence" (p. 754), seem to hold equally true for the therapist-supervisee as well as the supervisor.

Psychotherapy Training and Cultural Differences

The effort to reach a professional ideal and identity is a dynamic struggle through a therapist's residency years. Indeed, this period of time is also a journey of transition and apprenticeship. The years of apprenticeship are precisely those years during which occur what Erikson (1963) termed the process of intimacy versus isolation. Borrowing from Erikson's words, Levinson (1978) refers to the third and fourth decade of life as the "era of greatest contradiction and stress . . . [during which] one is struggling to establish his place in society" (p. 22). Within the training program of, for example, a university hospital, the trainee is placed in a hospital setting with other physicians and yet is simultaneously separate and different.

The vicissitudes of the struggle to become a psychiatrist or recognized therapist are intimately linked up not only with the process of studying for specialty or comprehensive exams and developing a diagnostic acumen but also with furthering a way of being and relating to self, colleagues, and patients. One of the most accessible real models and one of the most intimate and contributory relationships in psychotherapy training is the supervisory relationship. The supervisor may stand as a parental figure, in loco parentis: a mentor, a teacher, a disciplinarian, and a role model to the supervisee (Alonso 1985). Of the multiple functions that the supervisor may have, one of the most crucial at an early stage of the trainee's career is that of the figure with whom the trainee can identify. The trainee may identify with the character and ideals of the supervisor, the particular therapeutic approach the supervisor uses with patients, the supervisor's ways of interacting with colleagues and with others known in professional work and personal life, and particularly with the way the supervisor listens and responds to the supervisee's experience.

Alternatively, the supervisee from another culture may feel misunderstood, marginalized, responded to in an indifferent or prejudicial manner, and unable to express his or her particular perspectives. Cultural divergences may make the supervisee more vigilant and anxious about the supervisor's capacity to attend to and critically evaluate the supervisee's experience and performance. When the supervisee comes from a different country, speaks a different mother tongue, is a member of a racial or ethnic minority, and/or is of a different religion from the dominant culture supervisor, the capacity to identify with the supervisor may be made more difficult than with a colleague who shares similar or convergent cultural determinants.

External and internal conflicts related to acculturation can be complicated; the "foreign" supervisee may feel at risk of losing a vital sense of self, based on ethnocultural similarities with his or her culture of origin. On the other hand, the "foreign" supervisee may feel some relief in embracing a new culture, particularly if he or she has had to leave the home country for political, psychological, or social reasons. All too often, the supervisee from another culture may be a political refugee. Also, the supervisee may have had to abandon a previous career. As a result, he or she will be older, with competing demands (e.g., obtaining full licensing requirements, dealing with resettled parents and children, managing financial difficulties) that may obtrude on the supervision in many ways. The supervisor may face other tasks within the supervisory relationship, in addition to the traditional supervision of the psychotherapeutic work. He or she may be called upon to be more of a mentor, parent-like figure, or confidant: for example, the supervisee may share a passing domestic concern or doubt about his or her training. The supervisor is charged with the task of being available to the supervisee, not as a therapist investigating genetic or dynamic personal issues nor a patronizing figure, but as a responsive and respectful fellow professional who may offer some helpful direction. If the supervisor denies the extent of the supervisee's cultural difference, or fails to evaluate the way in which cultural differences may impinge on dynamic factors, the psychotherapy supervision may be adversely affected.

Impact of Cultural Difference

Wilkeson (1982), writing from the perspective of a Puerto Rican resident, noted that "the resident's own different cultural background was usually ignored by peers and supervisors while residents felt an implicit, strong expectation to reaffirm 'the white institution's concepts of itself as liberal, unbiased, and nondiscriminatory'" (p. 285). Varghese (1983) suggests that failure to appreciate the impact of racial difference can impede therapeutic progress, and such observations have implications for the supervisory process.

Reviewing four cases with a black supervisor and white super-visee, Remington and DaCosta (1989) describe how "failure to deal with these issues can adversely affect the supervisory relationship, the supervised therapy, and the overall education of the resident" (p. 398). Davidson (1987) wrote about her experiences as a psychother-apy supervisor in Japan and stressed the importance of "helping a supervisee keep his or her cultural identity while undergoing a 'West-ernizing identity diffusion'" (p. 234). Muslin and Val (1980) recom-mended entering the inner world of the student, yet noted that the "path to achieve this goal . . . with students who are at a great psy-chological distance from *one's self*, who are 'foreign' in habits, dress, gestures, and other patterns of communication has at times been full of obstacles" (p. 546). Holmes (1992) offers a caveat to therapists and supervisors dealing with cultural issues: she suggests that such coun-tertransferential possibilities deserve consideration within supervi-sion, as well as in the therapist's own therapy and ongoing self-analysis.

Sense of a Cultural Self

Volkan (1987) refers to the sense of self

[that] can be considered as a collection, both conscious and un-conscious, of perceptions and experiences of one's mind and body, and the feeling states attached to such perceptions and experiences . . . the sense of self, whether that of an individual or group, adheres more stubbornly than ever to a sense of ethnicity when stressed by a political crisis. (p. 906)

Moses (1982) describes the increase or decrease in self-esteem associated with the projection of bad aggressive impulses onto a scapegoat or external enemy. Such impulses may be projected by either participant in supervision or by the patient, or they may be triggered by sociopolitical crises outside the supervision.

A first-year inpatient psychiatric resident, a female foreign med-ical graduate (FMG), saw a Spanish-speaking woman from Colombia who had been repeatedly abused as a child and adult. The psychotherapeutic relationship between supervisee and patient was good; the inpatient, who was initially depressed, responded positively to supportive and empathic interventions by the resident. The resident appeared eager to please her supervisor and adopted a deferential manner as she presented her case. At the outset of supervision, the supervisor respectfully asked if they could discuss their cultural differences, because at some point this might influence their work together. The resident agreed and disclosed that she had grown up in a large town in Egypt and was from a religious minority; in return, the supervisor disclosed that he was Jewish and raised in North America.

The area of cultural difference did not come up in the supervisory relationship for some months, although the fact that the area had been broached in a neutral and introductory way allowed for some brief discussions. Cultural, legal, and psychological attitudes toward physical and sexual abuse to women were discussed in the therapy of the patient, as well as the prevailing cultural paternalism in the resident's country of origin. In the winter of 1991, an event of international magnitude occurred that raised considerable anxiety within the supervisory relationship. Alleged atrocities and hostilities leading up to the impasse between the United States, its allies, Israel, and Iraq had reached a crucial breaking point. The resident expressed her fears that "something terrible will happen."

The supervisor felt uneasy and reflected that the resident, an Egyptian, might experience some hostile remark in a predominantly Jewish hospital (i.e., Mount Sinai Hospital). Indeed, on one occasion another staffer assumed incorrectly that the resident was Muslim and asked her about her "countertransference." At this point, she expressed a pique of consternation and explained tearfully to her psychotherapy supervisor that she herself had experienced persecution in Egypt because she was not Muslim, but a minority within the Muslim majority.

This case illustrates some of the complexities in psychotherapy supervision when participants are from different cultures. The resident functioned effectively as a psychotherapist; in supervision, she tended to identify with the passive but resourceful female patient who had been abused by a family member. She did not discuss cultural differences with her other supervisors because this was never asked of her. Thus, they could not know the extent of her distress during the Persian Gulf crisis, nor her own experience of persecution.

During times of external or internal crisis, regressive experiences of the self may occur. In this instance, the spectre of uncontrolled aggression and consequent persecutory anxiety in a sensitive political area for both supervisor and supervisee could stimulate counterprojections of unacceptable hostile attitudes onto the "other." I suggest that cultural differences should be disclosed and discussed openly at the outset of supervision. Setting the stage for an acceptance and tolerance of difference may lead to a greater shared understanding as well as to the capacity of the supervisee to positively identify with the stable role of the supervisor. In this case, the resident and her supervisor were able to discuss their apprehension about the Gulf crisis and reveal each other's respective positions. Ethnocultural issues—religious, racial, linguistic—if not addressed or acknowledged, may serve to increase anxiety within the supervisory relationship.

Dimensions of Cultural Experience: Canada and the United States

One relevant cultural factor that may be examined is the number of physicians graduating from universities outside of Canada and the United States. In the province of Ontario, for example, of 17,535 active licensed physicians, 29% were foreign medical graduates (Ontario Physician Manpower Data Centre 1988). By specialty, 46% of Ontario's psychiatrists practice in the Metropolitan Toronto area. Of these, 34% were FMGs (Ontario Physician Manpower Data Centre 1989). These figures indicate that a substantial proportion of Toronto psychiatrists are trained in foreign medical universities and therefore have different ethnocultural and linguistic traditions.

It is estimated that half of all immigrants to Canada move to Ontario, and that approximately half of Ontario immigrants settle in

Metropolitan Toronto. Surveys from Statistics Canada show that up to 50% of the population of Metropolitan Toronto in 1987 was composed of persons whose first language was not English (E.S.L./D Work Group Report 1988). According to one university source, the percentage of FMG residents in the University of Toronto (U of T) postgraduate psychiatry program approximated 30% (D. Kussin, personal communication, April 1991). When comparing the number of FMG physicians in Ontario with the number of FMG psychiatrists in Metropolitan Toronto, and then the percentage of FMGs putatively enrolled in postgraduate psychiatry at U of T, it can be seen that a sizable amount—about 30%—reflects the proportion of FMGs in the total population of physicians, specialists, and residents. These data suggest that the area of cultural difference is a major phenomenon that has been insufficiently studied.

In the United States, Tarjan (1984), himself an FMG, has tersely written about his experience: "I was born and reared in Hungary, graduated from medical school there, came to the United States with no practical knowledge of English, and encountered the usual licensing problems" (p. 925).

Professional Underrepresentation of Cultural Groups

Tarjan (1984) points out that FMGs as a group represent about 25% of the membership of the American Psychiatric Association (APA) and 40% of the psychiatrists who work in public settings. Talbott (1984) has drawn attention to the underrepresentation of FMGs in the APA: "Over one-third of the candidates for the American Board of Psychiatry and Neurology's examination are FMGs, and their failure rate is eight times that of the U.S. medical graduates; although one-fourth of the APA members are FMGs, only a few serve on committees" (p. 929).

Petersdorf and colleagues (1990) estimated that the 1990 U.S. Census would show the population of the United States to be 13% black, 8% Hispanic, less than 1% Native American, and 2% Asian and Pacific Islander, totaling about 24%. Despite current efforts, Petersdorf and colleagues (1990) admit that for many years, American medical schools mirrored the discrimination of American society. Blacks, Native Americans, Mexican Americans, and mainland Puerto Ricans were underrepresented in medicine. The Association of American Medical Colleges (AAMC) Faculty Roster data base indicates that the proportion of minorities designated as underrepresented accounts for only 2.9% of faculty positions. What about the administrators and training directors whose responsibility it is to offer teaching in cultural psychotherapy and supervision and to increase the representation of cultural minorities in training programs? As Pinderhughes and Pinderhughes (1982) observed:

> Training directors and faculty members are less likely to be involved significantly in intercultural, interethnic, and interracial therapy than the residents they train. When faculty members speak positively of their private patients and only supervise but do not treat the public ward or clinic patients, residents are being trained in prejudices and patterns of discrimination that have been institutionalized in medical care for a long time. (p. 249)

Language

Language, the most accessible means of communicating meaning to others, also represents a key cultural element in the composition of ego identity. "Language is described as the most important and traditional aspect of a culture as well as the most resistant to change" (Freire 1991, p. 3).

▼ Linguistic Competence and Anxiety

A resident, a fully trained physician and a mother of young children, was forced to leave her repressive South American homeland and enter a psychiatric residency in Canada. She reported a dream from which she awoke in a state of panic. In the dream, she addressed a Spanish-speaking audience but delivered the speech in English. She overheard someone in the audience whispering: "Dr. X doesn't want to speak Spanish any longer." The resident woke up with a tremendous sense of vulnerability and fragmentation that stayed with her for several days. Following graduation from a psychiatry program, she wrote of her experience and those of other refugees and immigrants: "These people find the inability to communicate in the new language the most punitive aspect of their first encounter with the new society . . . in order to learn a second language the individual has to give up more of himself . . . along with native language the memories, feelings, emotions, and life experiences, identity itself may be gone. . . . "

"For years," she wrote, "I was surprised that people understood my verbalizations in English. I was able to put words and complex sentences in place, but the emotional connections had not yet been made. I only experienced the visual imagery, the flavor and the smell of it when I ate *manzana,* but not when I ate an apple. As a psychiatric resident, the statement, 'I am going to kill myself' would mobilize in me a number of practical responses leading to the proper management of the suicidal patient. It took one patient to say to me 'me voy a matar' to trigger the emotional response." (Freire 1990, p. 4)

The resident from another culture who appears to express him- or herself passably well may be still wrestling with uncertainties about acquisition of a second language, therapeutic competence, and doubts about self-regard and critical acceptance. A supervisory relationship offers not only didactic or technical interventions, but also an empathic and confirming presence to support an individual at a crucial state of development and training.

▼ Anxieties Over Competence and Acceptance

A Toronto-born second-year resident was affiliated with a francophone community psychiatry rotation in Montréal. He attended case conferences in both English and French, carried a case load of anglophone and francophone patients, and correspondingly had anglophone and francophone supervisors. With his anglophone supervisor, he felt at ease and relatively competent, and his level of anxiety did not seem to interfere with his capacity to attend and learn from the manifest and latent aspects of clinical material. However, when he met with his francophone supervisor, the resident felt himself to be uncertain and wondered if he fully understood the comments of his francophone supervisor and colleagues. Might they be downplaying or ridiculing what seemed to him to be his awkward case presentations? Dynamic issues appeared less clear with the resident's francophone cases, although his work was not subject to stringent criticism as he feared. On the other hand, he noted some difficulties of his francophone colleagues with anglophone supervisors and rounds. He found himself wincing at their faux pas, disconcerted and yet reassured that only a few residents were perfectly bilingual.

At night, on call, the resident had to check with francophone colleagues and even nursing supervisors for confirmation to make sure he had not committed any clinical errors of judgment. In the morning, he verified his work with secretaries so that his dictated French summaries made sense. From one service to the next, from one language to the next, he was struck by how greatly his self-esteem, anxiety, and self-consciousness altered. He marvelled at the stable felicity with which certain secretaries, nurses, physicians, and supervisors were able to consistently switch from one language and culture to another. The resident's francophone supervisor appeared as an empathic and reassuring figure, offering encouragement and affiliation.

This resident, by dint of his rotation as a "cultural minority" in a francophone community psychiatry program, was able to intimately experience a profound alteration in his sense of self, competency, and affective state. Through these cultural and linguistic transformations, although temporary, he began to appreciate what Freire (1990) has termed "'regressive position' of not being able to communicate in the new language . . . a reaffirmation of the regressive state of dependency and increased vulnerability . . . " (p. 5).

▼ Difficulty in Finding a Suitable Case

A male Asian FMG preresident was well known to the nurses because of the long hours he devoted to his inpatients. He appeared to diligently search for a suitable psychotherapy case without success. His psychotherapy supervisor offered papers on psychotherapy and arranged for him to see patients; but despite a number of referrals, the resident was unable to find a suitable psychotherapy case. After some months, the psychotherapy supervisor was impatient and concerned that the resident was in a supervisory impasse, because he was not involved in continuing psychotherapy with a patient. The supervisor was aware as well of his own pressing narcissistic needs to succeed with this resident, and he felt perplexed that the resident did not seem very interested in reading the psychotherapy literature. As time went on, however, the resident described himself more openly in the supervisory relationship and disclosed feelings related to difficulties with inpatients, frustrations with the racial biases of certain staff members, problems in training in a new country, and hopes of obtaining a medical license and earning financial independence. Soon after, he was able to engage a young depressed man in therapy.

The supervisor found himself in a dilemma. Was the resident's reluctance to find a suitable therapy case and read relevant literature an example of learning resistance and supervisory impasse? Or was it, rather, the outward manifestation of the apprehension of a young trainee who recently began a training program and needed his own time to attend to and approach issues relevant to his own development? By taking a more authoritative (or punitive) and didactic position, the supervisor believed he would risk losing the trust and openness of the resident. The supervisor elected a wait-and-see approach, nevertheless keeping the supervisory sessions available and open.

▼ A Resident Accused of Incompetence

A female FMG European physician in a preresidency position professed apprehension about her lack of knowledge of psychiatric diagnosis and psychotherapy. She followed a number of extremely difficult patients with character disorders and was quite disturbed when she was accused of being "no good," "the worst," and virtually "incompetent" by an angry borderline patient. The trainee expressed doubts about her linguistic abilities, her obvious accent, and her competence, and she was shaken by the patient's accusations and her countertransference reactions.

Supervision was directed at reflecting back to the resident evidence of her competence. The resident was able to "see" the devaluative defensive splitting and idealization that the patient used within the transference. The supervisor acknowledged the resident's preoccupation with linguistic factors and allowed her sense of "foreignness" to enter into the supervisory relationship. The supervisor disclosed a personal anecdote, illustrating that no matter how senior one was, there were difficulties in working with such patients. Some months later, the trainee laughingly reported that the same patient mentioned that she had been one of her best therapists. In later sessions, she described how she had recently attended lectures by two expert psychoanalytic therapists and noted, with pleasure, that despite their thick European accents, they were nevertheless experts in their field.

Working with psychotic patients who have character disorders is extremely trying for first-year residents, particularly when they come from different cultural backgrounds. Projective denigration and "scapegoating" of such residents by patients may threaten a struggling sense of trust, self-esteem, and competence, complicated by linguistic and cultural factors.

It is common knowledge that many first-year psychiatry residents and preresidents are placed on inpatient units with heightened exposure to acutely disturbed psychotic patients and patients with character disorders. Under these circumstances, adequate supervision is essential to deal with the sense of apprehension, isolation, and vulnerability the resident feels when exposed to patients who devalue, criticize, and direct negative split-off affect toward them.

Conclusion

Psychotherapy supervision is an interactive learning process between the psychotherapy supervisor and the supervisee. It can be thought of as operating on two separate levels: didactic/content and process/experiential. The first level implies a focus on teaching objective knowledge with a clear boundary between teacher and student. The implicit assumption is that the teacher is in the superior position as the unquestioned authority, and the student is in the inferior position as the uncertain apprentice. The second level implies a less hierarchical interaction in which the supervisee discusses his or her work with the supervisor and both attempt to understand each other's experiences. Clinical supervisory practice suggests that the supervisee (resident) from another culture is in a particularly vulnerable situation because of ethnocultural differences. If no supervisory attention is paid to these differences, the resident may find him- or herself in a misalliance—feeling misunderstood and unable to participate in supervision. Too strong an emphasis on a didactic approach may skew the supervisee toward viewing the supervisor as a critical and punitive authority, and the supervisee as inadequate and prone to failure.

This obviously discourages open communication of supervisee experience. Using a more expressive process-oriented model offers crucial regulatory feedback between supervisor and supervisee. This type of communication may enhance the developmental capacity of the supervisee from another culture at a crucial phase of his or her training program and lead to positive rather than negative identification with authority figures. In addition, this approach enables the supervisor from a different culture to reflect and compare his or her experience with that of the supervisee or patient. Given the heterogeneous nature of contemporary society, it is not unusual for patient, therapist, supervisor, and administrator to come from divergent cultures, yet be expected to join together in the process of psychotherapy and psychotherapy supervision.

I suggest that the administrator or director of a psychotherapy program has an influential and organizing role at the apex of the clinical rhombus. The director is in a position to implement cross-cultural teaching in the training curriculum, heighten supervisory awareness of cultural determinants, and serve as a leader and facilitator of further study and research.

References

Alonso A: The Quiet Profession: Supervisors of Psychotherapy. New York, Macmillan, 1985

Arlow JA: The supervisory situation. J Am Psychoanal Assoc 11:576–594, 1963

Brantley T: Racism and its impact on psychotherapy. Am J Psychiatry 140:1605–1608, 1983

Cavenar J, Spaulding JG: When the psychotherapist is black. Am J Psychiatry 135:1084–1087, 1978

Collins W: English Dictionary. London, William Collins & Sons, 1984

Davidson L: Supervision of psychotherapy east and west. Am J Psychoanal 47:230–236, 1987

Ekstein R, Wallerstein RS: The Teaching and Learning of Psychotherapy, 2nd Edition. New York, International Universities Press, 1972

Erikson E: Childhood and Society, 2nd Edition. New York, WW Norton, 1963

Fischer N: An interracial analysis: transference and countertransference significance. J Am Psychoanal Assoc 19:736–745, 1971

Foulks EF: The concept of culture in psychiatric residency education. Am J Psychiatry 137:811–816, 1980

Freire M: Refugees: ESL and literacy: trying to reinvent the self in a new language. Refuge 10(2):3–6, 1990

Freire M: Immigrant and refugee children: native language as a factor in the development of the self and the competent acquisition of a second language. Paper presented at the Immigrant and Refugee Children's Mental Health Research Symposium, Toronto, Ontario, February 1991

Holmes DE: Race and transference in psychoanalysis and psychotherapy. Int J Psychoanal 73:1–11, 1992

Jacques E: Social systems as defenses against persecutory and depressive anxiety, in New Directions in Psycho-Analysis. Edited by Klein M, Heimann P, Money-Kyrle R. London, Tavistock, 1955, pp 478–498

Levinson DJ: The Seasons of a Man's Life. New York, Ballantine Books, 1978

Moses R: The group self and the Arab-Israeli conflict. International Review of Psychoanalysis 9:55–65, 1982

Muslin H, Val E: Supervision and self-esteem in psychiatric teaching. Am J Psychother 34:545–555, 1980

Myers WA: Some issues involved in the supervision of interracial and transcultural treatments, in New Concepts in Psychoanalytic Psychotherapy. Edited by Ross JM, Myers WA. Washington, DC, American Psychiatric Press, 1988, pp 140–148

Obendorf CP: Selectivity and option for psychiatry. Am J Psychiatry 110:745–758, 1954

Ontario Physician Manpower Data Centre: Data on number of physicians graduating from universities outside Canada and United States (psychiatric specialists, place of graduation). Toronto, ON, Ontario Physician Manpower Data Centre, 1988 [address information requests for this and next reference to: The Ontario Physician Manpower Data Centre, Banting Institute, 100 College Street, Room 510, Toronto, ON, Canada M5G 1L5; tel. (416) 978-6720; fax (416) 978-6499]

Ontario Physician Manpower Data Centre: Data on specialty physician geographic location (physician registry, active physicians in Metropolitan Toronto). Toronto, ON, Ontario Physician Manpower Data Centre, 1989

Petersdorf RG, Turner KS, Nickens HW, et al: Minorities in medicine: past, present and future. Acad Med 65:663–670, 1990

Pinderhughes CA, Pinderhughes EB: Perspectives of the training directors, in Cross-Cultural Psychiatry. Edited by Gaw A. Boston, MA, John Wright, 1982, pp 247–286

Remington G, DaCosta G: Ethnocultural factors in resident supervision: black supervisor and white supervisees. Am J Psychother 43:398–404, 1989

Schacter JS, Butts HF: Transference and countertransference in interracial analysis. J Am Psychoanal Assoc 16:792–808, 1968

Talbott JA: Response to the presidential address: Psychiatry's unfinished business in the 20th century. Am J Psychiatry 141:927–928, 1984

Tarjan G: Presidential address—American psychiatry: a dynamic mosaic. Am J Psychiatry 141:923–927, 1984

Varghese FI: The racially different psychiatrist—implications for psychotherapy. Aust N Z J Psychiatry 17:329–333, 1983

Volkan V: Psychological concepts useful in building of political foundations between nations: track II diplomacy. J Am Psychoanal Assoc 35:903–936, 1987

Wilkeson AG: A resident's perspective, in Cross-Cultural Psychiatry. Edited by Gaw A. Boston, MA, John Wright, 1982, pp 285–299

Chapter 5

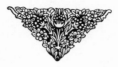

Supervision of the Beginning Psychiatric Resident

Stefan P. Stein, M.D.

Supervision is recognized as the cornerstone of clinical education in psychiatric residency training. This is true not only in the teaching of formal psychotherapy, but also in training in skills of assessment, principles of hospital management, and work with families and groups—essentially all clinical encounters. The goal of these supervisions is the development of a range of clinical skills essential for the psychiatric practitioner, whatever subspecialty he or she may choose.

How does supervision of the beginning resident in psychiatry facilitate this developmental learning process? In the context of an ongoing relationship between trainee and supervisor, the study of the care of patients provides opportunity for the resident to develop clinical skills and knowledge, accompanied by the evolution of the resident's self-concept from that of new medical doctor to that of a nascent psychiatrist.

Much attention has been directed to the study of the supervisory relationship, to the theory of supervision, and to the understanding of the vicissitudes of the supervisory alliance in relation to the therapy being supervised (Arlow 1963; Ekstein and Wallerstein 1972; Fleming and Benedek 1966; Grotjahn 1955). There has been less focus on the special problems of the supervision of the beginning psychiatric trainee, the area I will address in this chapter.

The Beginning Resident—From Medicine to Psychiatry

Residents are socialized into clinical medicine through a series of clerkships during the final 2 years of medical education. Clinical training in medical school is largely centered on the hospital treatment of severely ill patients. Students often train in tertiary care inpatient hospital facilities, with diffusion of responsibility for patients the norm. A "team" of three to five medical students and house staff physicians often cares for a patient, in addition to subspecialists, consultants, and a private attending physician. The patient's illness is at the center of the student's and resident's focus. The goal of care is defined as the reduction or elimination of "pathology." There is relatively little concern for the general state of the patient, apart from the specific medicopathological condition. Concern about personal elements in the patient's life is eschewed, especially if the patient has a chronic or fatal illness.

The medical armamentarium, symbolized by stethoscope and cards with "data" about the patient in the pocket of a white coat, distinguishes the student and young physician from the patient. Students model the house staff's disengagement from the patient.

The modal response to painful affects (e.g., anxiety, anger, or depression) that arise in working with the medical patient is avoidance. Helplessness, a particularly painful affect in relation to the physician's common fantasy of being a savior, is likewise warded off by denial and avoidance. The young doctor sees him- or herself as proactive, joined with fellow doctors in an effort to conquer illness. First-year experiences for psychiatric residents typically include at least 6 months of training on such acute medical and neurological services.

Psychiatric training, especially supervision, must revive affective availability in the period immediately following this medical experience. Training should encourage the development of different skills necessary for psychiatric diagnosis and treatment, in the context of deeper and more complex relationships with the patient. The beginning resident must learn to listen and understand, to empathize without becoming overwhelmed by the patient's distress and neediness, and to tolerate the patient's upset and anger without acting immediately to suppress them. Later, the development of specific psychotherapeutic skills follows as a goal for training.

Residents thus often begin psychiatric training after an orientation to medicine from the above-described perspective, without knowledge of the subtle aspects of the doctor/patient relationship. They may have little awareness of the meanings of transference and countertransference, or of other parameters of obvious or subtle aspects of the treatment situation. They are often unfamiliar with the model of supervision itself—how it functions, and what it can accomplish.

Residents have had varied prior psychiatry experience as medical students. For example, students may have worked only in an outpatient setting, or on a consultation liaison service, and may never have had any opportunity to become familiar with inpatients. There is a tendency for beginning residents to generalize, based on their limited experience, especially in the absence of other specific knowledge and under the impact of the stress of beginning work with severely ill psychiatric patients.

The beginning resident is usually assigned to a psychiatric inpatient service where he or she works with other mental health professionals, such as nurses, aides, psychologists, and social workers, who are more knowledgeable about the operation of a psychiatric unit and are more experienced in caring for patients. Although graduate physicians, residents are beginners in psychiatry. They are often reminded of their ignorance and lack of experience by permanent ward staff, who may resent the repeated task of "breaking in" new residents. The residents are often disheartened about their lack of competence and knowledge and may be particularly vulnerable to narcissistic injury from senior teachers and supervisors.

Residents consequently begin their training with highly varied backgrounds ranging from little or no experience to a few months of inpatient expertise, often without much specific information to orient them to clinical and didactic psychiatric problems apart from their medical identity. Under the impact of the stress in shifting to a new and strange setting (for them), they may manifest maladaptive or defensive behaviors in their beginning work. Supervision provides critical early assistance in this difficult period.

I am assuming that training takes place in a program structured around the biopsychosocial model of treatment on a general inpatient service. The supervision discussed in this chapter is often provided by an "off unit" supervisor who works individually with the resident. The goal of this supervision is to help the resident develop beginning skills in evaluation, formulation, and "psychotherapeutic" exchanges with the patient, in contrast with the supervision of formal ongoing psychotherapy.

The importance of the unit director's role in setting the overall educational mission cannot be overemphasized. Although my discussion focuses on the role of individual supervision, it is highly desirable that the entire staff assist the resident in identifying educational questions. The unit chief ideally renews the staff's interest and commitment to education as a mission for all professionals, which at times may be displaced by the pressing tasks of clinical care. The role of the nurses, in particular, can be critical. Day-to-day clinical decisions about patients' statuses, passes, and other issues can become learning experiences that residents bring into supervision, rather than "disposition" matters to be decided by the "treatment team."

The tasks of a resident on such a service are complex and include those of the "responsible physician" who writes orders, manages medication, and (with others on the staff, as noted previously) decides about passes and discharge planning. The resident performs a physical examination, is responsible for the patient's medical management, and provides general medical care during the patient's stay.

This multidimensional "real" relationship requires that the resident interact with the patient across a wide range of activity. The removed quality that characterizes defined psychotherapy is thus not possible given these other tasks. Nonetheless, residents can learn to listen with a psychodynamically tuned ear for underlying themes in the material the patient presents, and they can learn to recognize transference and countertransference manifestations that enter the treatment relationship. Residents also have the opportunity to learn about the effects of hospitalization and other treatment interventions on the level of regression, and about other shifts in the patient's defensive structure evident in thought and behavior. In addition, residents learn to be "therapeutic." The resident who can clarify a preconscious affective state for a patient, for example, may help the patient to feel better understood and may develop the basis for a treatment that includes more in-depth psychotherapy, if indicated. The resident should come to understand from firsthand experience that to help a patient feel understood in a new way can be highly supportive for the patient, and this may facilitate an improved doctor-patient relationship for the entire treatment.

Responses of Residents to Beginning Work on a Psychiatric Service

Ornstein (1968) described the Sorcerer's Apprentice phenomenon in residents' early work with patients: residents often see supervisors' and other faculty's clinical behavior as powerful, in a magical way. They may imitate the behavior without understanding its framework, the reasons for its use, or the factors that make it effective.

> A beginning resident observed his unit chief confront a patient at a community meeting. This senior psychiatrist tactfully told the patient that he (the patient) was angry and needed to regain control. The resident became anxious, fearing that the patient, who was psychotic and had been assaultive, might attack others on the unit. The resident thereafter reported to his supervisor, a psychoanalyst, that he (the resident) was concerned about one of his patients. He explained that he had "confronted" the patient, a man about the same age as the resident, regarding "his hostility," in an ill conceived attempt to diffuse his own anxiety. The magic of "confrontation" was misused, resulting in the patient becoming angry and refusing to talk to the resident. Bewildered and anxious, the resident continued to attempt to "interpret" to the patient, in an "analytic mode," the patient's anger as having its source in his relationship to his father.

This illustration underlines the element of caricature that is sometimes evident in the resident's early work with patients. Other common patterns include extreme passivity, imitating the fantasized "analytic neutrality" of psychoanalysis. The opposite attitude may also be present—that of a resident's believing that he or she can quickly "analyze" all that troubles the patient, or, finally, a total denigration of "talking therapy." Residents may also believe that they must meet with every patient for 45-minute sessions (the "correct" therapy hour) regardless of the patient's clinical condition and of other parameters of treatment, such as length of hospital stay.

The beginning resident often comes to the first supervisory hour without an understanding of the fundamental principles of the work he or she is to do (i.e., a mixture of patient evaluation, hospital management, and planning and implementation of a complex treatment program). In addition, the resident often lacks the capacity to simply sit with and listen to the patient, creating the conditions in which the patient can tell his or her story. He or she often works psychotherapeutically with the patient in a manner largely determined or modified by his or her own defensive needs.

The Initial Phase of Supervision

Fleming (1953) described phases of learning in supervision of residents. The first phase is characterized by "imitative learning." She observed the danger of mechanical imitation similar to that described by Ornstein (1968). Grotjahn (1949) spoke of identification in supervision "done out of anxiety" as providing protection from the fear of being like the patient; "it is less anxiety-causing to be a doctor than to be a patient." Identification is a valuable and even essential aspect of the long course of learning the techniques of psychotherapy. But the anxious surroundings, lack of experience, and paucity of theoretical knowledge of the beginning trainee combine to create a setting in which identifications may assume the quality of caricature or superficial imitation, not integrated into a larger whole.

A major determinant of the fate of the beginning resident's initial encounters with patients is his or her experience with supervisors. Although much attention is directed by the ward staff to management decisions (e.g., somatic therapies, patient status, and passes), there is often a lack of attention to the "talking" therapeutic contact between resident and patient. The often bewildered resident is told that "formal" psychotherapy is not indicated or possible, yet the resident knows that he or she must talk and (one hopes) listen to the patient. The supervisor thus faces the difficult task of supervising a special talking therapy, conducted by an anxious beginner, managing severely ill patients.

Supervising the beginning resident requires a flexible model that takes into account the beginning level of the supervisee. It may encompass an informal didactic component as well as direct supervisory experience, and it should be guided by an awareness of the major impact that early identification with the supervisor may have.

Suggested General Principles

The supervisor must be prepared to shift modes from listening for the resident's basic difficulties in meeting with the patient, to responding to the resident's lack of capacity to develop a comprehensive formulation of the patient's psychopathology as a treatment framework, to responding to the need to attend to dynamic themes as well as the manifest content.

> A male resident who was single reported to a supervisor that an acutely psychotic and physically attractive female patient had asked his age and marital status. He anxiously explained to the supervisor that he could not answer her because he felt she was being "seductive." He knew no way to respond other than silence, if he was not to "play into her hand."
>
> The supervisor responded by helping him think through a series of possible meanings the patient's question might have, emphasizing an understanding of her distress, isolation, low self-esteem, and ego disturbances. He suggested that the resident had several options, each of which would have different consequences for his work with the patient. The resident listened at-

tentively and expressed relief that there were not only systematic approaches to assessing the situation and to organizing a response, but also that there was no single "right" way. The supervisor presented models for the resident that considered these issues:

1. Awareness of the patient's distress and overall mental state;
2. A learning, listening attitude in the treatment directed at understanding inner as well as manifest meanings for the patient; and
3. A model suggesting that there often is no one correct response in a given clinical situation.

The presentation of several approaches to understanding the patient's question and a number of possible responses was critical for this resident. Rather than a silent, "nonresponsive" or omnipotent master, the resident experienced a thoughtful, empathic (to him), active listener and physician-psychiatrist who used psychodynamic principles in working with a psychotic inpatient.

The supervisor must be prepared to work with beginning residents at levels of knowledge and skill varying from absolute novice to relatively experienced. It is strongly recommended that the supervisor spend the first hour inquiring about the trainee's previous experience and his or her general familiarity with psychopathology, psychological concepts and treatment models, and nature of supervision itself. This will also help the resident develop trust and will lead to the development of the supervisory alliance, which is necessary if maximal learning is to occur.

Beginning residents frequently have had no experience in working with a supervisor on a regular basis over a period of time. They are often uncertain about the propriety of disclosure, and they may fear that the supervisor might see them as ill if they reveal personal issues that arise in the course of the supervision. The supervisor's willingness to reveal experiences he or she has had in clinical work may be helpful in teaching the resident that intense personal reactions to patients are not only common but in fact may be extremely useful in the diagnostic and therapeutic process. In addition to relieving the beginning resident's anxiety about reactions he or she may be having, disclosure of such experiences by a supervisor provides a model for learning to use these reactions in the supervisory process, and ultimately in the treatment of the patient.

Not all faculty are well equipped to supervise beginning residents. Some may not be familiar with the current organization and needs of inpatient services or may feel unqualified to supervise the care of severely ill inpatients. The program director should carefully select for this task those faculty who have personal and professional qualities required for work with beginning residents.

Early sessions are important in helping residents to learn the skills of clinical assessment, as well as the need to listen for themes, to identify psychodynamic issues by integrating historical information, and to use information from the "here and now" of the interview. In this way, the beginning resident develops a framework for understanding and organizing clinical psychopathological and psychological data. Occasional suggestions for related readings may be useful to help the beginner develop models for conceptualizing the specifics with which he or she is dealing.

A major pitfall in early clinical work lies in the frequent confusion between the psychological theories of psychoanalysis (i.e., psychodynamic psychology and the techniques of psychoanalytic treatment per se). Beginning residents may misconstrue a supervisor's efforts in developing psychodynamic *understanding* of clinical material as a mandate to behave with the patient in an overly "psychoanalytic" mode. The likelihood of this confusion is increased if the supervisor assumes an "analytic" style of listening in the supervision.

Interviewing the patient, together with the resident, is often critical in the supervision of beginning residents. A joint interview of a patient (led off by the resident and, in a planned way, completed by the supervisor) allows the supervisor to directly observe the resident's clinical work and thus comment in a practical and cogent way. It provides an opportunity for modeling by the resident and allows the supervisor to comment on the patient in a way not possible with the sometimes inaccurate data of a beginner's reporting. The joint interview also establishes collegiality and demystifies the supervisor. Watching a supervisor struggle to interview an angry, paranoid patient is helpful and reassuring to a beginner who is concerned about his or her very suitability for psychiatry based on difficulties in beginning clinical work.

Early work with residents treating severely ill inpatients requires a responsive supervisor, alert to the resident's total response to the patient. This includes both that which is apparent to the resident, and that which appears in the supervisory relationship as enactment or other transference-like phenomena. However, the beginner is frequently unable to "hear" comments that refer to his or her intrapsychic processes. The supervisor must work sensitively to alert the resident, first, to the importance of psychological forces outside conscious awareness in the treatment and the supervision itself, and later, to direct attention to the need for ongoing self-examination, which will enable the resident to use the inner reactions to better inform the treatment. Psychodynamic data from the supervision will help this process later in the supervision.

Early difficulties in the resident's work may have many sources. The failure of empathy is best thought of as an issue only after other educational matters have been considered. The beginning resident's anxiety and apparent lack of empathy are often a response to a severely ill patient's dyscontrol, distress, or demands. The resident who has not learned how to respond to the patient is far more likely to distance him- or herself from the patient and appear "nonempathic" than is the better-informed beginner helped to resolve inner distress by a responsive senior colleague who is nonpunitive in attitude and able to accommodate to the inexperience and ignorance of the beginner.

The unresponsive supervisor is often experienced as critical, awesome, and out of touch with the trainee's work and struggles. As the resident must deal with both real and psychological issues in working with patients who have major ego deficits, so must the supervisor be attentive to the full range of issues in the supervisee. In sum, the supervisor must be particularly aware of the fact that he or she is supervising a beginning trainee, rather than only the care of a particular patient.

Later, work with the resident can begin to address process issues in the supervision and the treatment. Supervisors may also help residents to conceptualize how different types of psychotherapy may or may not be useful for particular patients. Later in the year, residents may, with the supervisor's help, identify selected patients for whom more intensive psychotherapy may be indicated during the inpatient stay. These patients may then be treated with scheduled, structured, dynamically oriented brief psychotherapy, while other more disorganized patients may be seen briefly on a daily basis with supportive treatment as the model.

Supervision of the patients selected for psychotherapy will provide an opportunity for directing attention to the process issues of both the treatment and the supervision. Psychotherapy per se becomes distinguished from psychodynamically informed hospital management, and the resident will work toward the development of the necessary skills required for this modality.

If there is a more structured psychotherapy later in the year, residents may be taught the use of process notes, introducing these beginning psychotherapists to the concept of data in supervision, in addition to simple recall. Other techniques, including use of videotape and audiotape, may be introduced as well. The supervisor is then able to listen to reports or recordings of sessions and comments on a broad range of issues, including the emergence of themes in the material, the nature of the transference and countertransference (where relevant), and the presence of blind spots and other defensive aspects of the resident's work. The supervision will have succeeded in encouraging the resident's growth from anxious outsider to functioning junior colleague.

Summary

Supervision of the beginning resident requires a flexible and responsive supervisor. It should incorporate aspects of the roles of clinical teacher and tutor and avoid the model of "master" and "analyst," in their omnipotent and omniscient sense. Above all, it requires flexibility, responsiveness, and a willingness to include interviewing a patient or discussing events on the unit that may be confusing or upsetting to the resident. A model that presents alternative approaches to understanding the patient, or to making interventions, is particularly useful.

References

Arlow J: The supervisory situation. J Am Psychoanal Assoc 11:576–594, 1963

Ekstein R, Wallerstein RS: The Teaching and Learning of Psychotherapy, 2nd Edition. New York, International Universities Press, 1972

Fleming J: The role of supervision in psychiatric training. Bull Menninger Clin 17(5):157–169, 1953

Fléming J, Benedek T: Psychoanalytic Supervision. New York, Grune & Stratton, 1966

Grotjahn M: The role of identification in psychiatry and psychoanalytic training. Psychiatry 12:141–151, 1949

Grotjahn M: Problems and technique of supervision. Psychiatry 18:9–15, 1955

Ornstein PH: Sorcerer's apprentice: the initial phase of training and education in psychiatry. Compr Psychiatry 9:293–315, 1968

Chapter 6

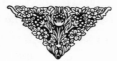

The Supervisee's Experience of Supervision

Jon Hunter, M.D., F.R.C.P.C., and
Debra A. Pinsky, M.D.

Psychotherapy supervision remains the keystone of learning about psychotherapy for resident trainees. It may be the highlight of their week. Rather than rushing around to fill out forms, find beds, or sit in endless meetings, residents have a chance to discuss with experienced teachers the intense and often valued time spent with their psychotherapy patients. The hope is to gain knowledge, insight, and capability. Yet supervision may be perceived as a time of scrutiny by an unfriendly observer—which may make it a time to be avoided or kept within manageable bounds by the selective "reconstruction" of the therapy sessions under review.

Obviously, the goal of psychotherapy supervision is not just resident satisfaction. However, in keeping with Rice and Fey's (1970) proposal, it seems that "the student's sense of satisfaction with [the] instructor may offer a natural and direct measure of his teaching effectiveness" (p. 174). Therefore, an examination of what psychiatric residents and other trainees rank as satisfying about this specific form of instruction may provide important insight into how to increase the educational value of a psychotherapy supervision.

What makes for a successful supervisory experience from the point of view of the resident? The literature on this question, albeit sparse, lends itself to a certain categorization. There is the innate importance of the match between the trainee and the supervisor, but there are also certain identifiable qualities that make the supervision useful. These characteristics can be divided into the following questions, which address three domains of the supervisory experience from the resident's perspective.

1. Who is the supervisor? What is the identity or what are the personality characteristics of successful supervisors?
2. What does the supervisor do? What is the content of supervision?
3. How does the supervisor do it? What is the process of supervision?

Each of these questions (given a certain degree of overlap) is examined in turn.

Who Is the Supervisor?

A number of studies have looked at the supervisory process, and some of these have elicited how trainees (psychiatric and others) have described their best supervisors. Nelson (1978) asked 48 trainees from various disciplines to pick preferences of opposing supervisory characteristics. He found that flexible, self-revealing, and permissive qualities were chosen. Miller and Oetting (1966) found that, with respect to the supervisor's personality, a good experience was commensurate with a "nonthreatening, tactful, nonauthoritarian" supervisor, whereas a bad experience occurred with supervisors who were "biased, rigid, domineering, and defensive." In interviews with residents, Kraft Goin and Kline (1974) noted that they expressed appreciation for the supervisors' respectful attitude.

The other crucial factor perhaps often taken for granted is that the resident wants and expects the supervisor to be an expert. In Pate and Wolff's (1990) study of 36 residents at Baylor University, the supervisor's ability to teach, capacity to establish rapport, and fund of knowledge were the three qualities ranked highest. The supervisor whose only continuing interest in psychotherapy occurs through the supervision of one or two cases per year is often experienced as a kind of dilettante who is just "keeping a hand in," thereby acquiring the status of a supervisor inappropriately. Alternatively, the experienced practitioner who conveys immediately the sense of sharing these issues on a day-to-day basis is not only tolerated but often sought after, no matter how irascible he or she may be, as suggested by Gale (1976).

Supervisors are expected to be expert teachers as well as expert clinicians. In a survey of Canadian psychiatric residents by Perez and colleagues (1984), "general teaching ability" and "ability to pinpoint residents' psychotherapy shortcomings and a willingness to help residents overcome them" (p. 658) received very high ratings.

This is also reflected in Shanfield and Gil's (1985) study on supervisory style. They delineate four main styles of supervisors: 1) facilitative, 2) confrontative and directive, 3) expert, and 4) task oriented. From their study, Shanfield and Gil found that most supervisors use predominantly one style and that residents will respond differently to each style. In general, it is believed that even an increased awareness of one style can improve supervisory effectiveness.

Taken in total, these data show that residents have a positive experience in psychotherapy supervision when a supervisor is an expert therapist and teacher who is able to provide direct feedback and information. The data also demonstrate that the personal attributes of being nonauthoritarian, nonthreatening, respectful, tactful, flexible, and permissive are paramount in providing a basic positive framework for supervision.

What Does the Supervisor Do?

What supervisors do or the content of the supervision has often been put forward as the crucial educational element. Although having only five supervisor-supervisee pairs in their sample, Kraft Goin and Kline (1974) looked specifically at what types of comments differentiated higher- versus lower-ranked supervisors in this regard.

Their results illustrate that the highly ranked supervisors more frequently (i.e., 15% and 21% versus 2%, 5%, and 9%) directed interventions to "information giving comments about technique." In fact, the
residents thought that more than 50% of the excellent supervisors'
helpful comments were about the techniques or principles of psychotherapy.

Perez and colleagues (1984) noted that, with roughly 160 respondents to their survey, the top 3 elements of supervision in descending
order of importance were assessment of patients (80.8%), understanding of a patient's psychodynamic aspects (77%), and formulation of treatment approach (74.5%). Perez and colleagues also found
that residents believed that formulation of treatment approach and
goals as well as techniques of transferring patients and termination
of therapy were usually dealt with inadequately, despite their importance. This suggests that what excellent supervisors say has to do
with what technique or principle of psychotherapy assessment and
management may be most relevantly applied to the present clinical
situation. Quotations from the residents in the Kraft Goin and Kline
(1974) study emphasize the excellent supervisor's capacity to reveal
"the theme" and "present a theoretical framework" (p. 212) that
guides interpretations.

In a confirmatory study, Kline and colleagues (1977) performed
content analysis of videotapes of supervision. They found that the
more highly rated supervisors focused on transference, understanding the dynamics of patients, and understanding the process between
patient and therapist. They did this while remaining in touch with
the central therapeutic problems. The factor analysis suggested that
supervisors who talk about things in general also tend to talk about
themselves and not focus on the specific work with the patient, leading to less resident satisfaction. However, they noted that "undoubtedly appropriate clinical examples are helpful."

In fact, there is one kind of clinical example that is much more
than just helpful. It is the anecdote in which the supervisor has not
had a striking success, but has faced a problem or failure. This disclosure conveys several important things simultaneously. Primarily it
clarifies that a therapist of the supervisor's stature is not perfect but
rather "good enough." Second, it reduces the distance between su-

pervisor and supervisee and emphasizes that such failures or miscues are a normal part of "growing up" professionally. This makes the resident's task of acquiring psychotherapeutic ability less daunting. Third, it models self-disclosure for the resident and encourages examination and discussion of those things that feel like failures, which are often the hardest to reveal within psychotherapy supervision. Therefore, the supervisors who appropriately self-disclose about failures are probably not the same supervisors who miss the mark by "talking about themselves and things in general." Rather, they have empathically appreciated a resident's anxiety, embarrassment, or shame and are able to defuse it by acknowledging similar experience or traits within themselves. As Markson and colleagues stated:

> The supervisor's willingness to speak of his own technical and theoretical quandaries is most helpful. He should be able to tolerate ignorance, ambiguity, impotence, failure, and all the painful experiences which a therapist must be capable of enduring. This is most helpful to the beginning psychotherapist who is so often inclined to expect far too much both from himself and his patient. (Greben et al. 1973, p. 475)

In essence, one vital aspect of what a supervisor does is provide a role model for the trainee. It is crucial to be aware that the trainee will look to the supervisor for his or her actions as well as words. In this way, a supervisor can easily model the qualities necessary to become an effective therapist. From the beginning of a supervisory relationship, the supervisor is given the opportunity to demonstrate the skills of negotiating the contract of a professional relationship that can then be converted, for the trainee, into the parallel techniques of negotiating a therapeutic relationship. Enabling the relationship to tolerate open and honest communication from the beginning serves as an experiential teaching tool for the trainee. Additionally, it gives permission to address in the future any glitches that occur within the supervisor-supervisee relationship that may provide further clues to what is happening in the therapy with the patient.

This way of understanding what a supervisor says actually implies the significance of how it is said or the process component of the supervision.

How Does the Supervisor Do It?

Supervisors' actions (or more accurately, interactions) refer to the process that occurs between supervisee and supervisor. The importance of establishing a rapport is reflected in its repeated emphasis in all studies. Perez and colleagues (1984) and Pate and Wolff (1990) report rapport as being within the top three most desired characteristics of supervision. Kline and colleagues (1977; Kraft Goin and Kline 1974) refer to the necessity of "a feeling of emotional involvement" with the resident and the treatment as well as the resident's "appreciation for the respectful attitude and rapport that was easily established" (Kraft Goin and Kline 1974, p. 212) by the supervisor. Those supervisors who cannot usually create an atmosphere of rapport (and therefore safety) for the resident are unlikely to be experienced as good or helpful and probably never get "out of the blocks" in the supervisory relationship.

Perhaps one of the crucial factors involved in establishing rapport is the recognition of the developmental stage of the particular resident in his or her acquisition of knowledge about psychotherapy. A resident (depending on his or her personal capacity, experience, and interest) wants or requires various kinds of supervision or knowledge at different stages of training. Perhaps the very first knowledge required is about the supervisory process itself. For the novice resident, supervision is an unknown event about which certain fantasies exist. At the Massachusetts Mental Health Center, Pinsky and colleagues developed a one-time didactic exercise for all incoming residents (D. A. Pinsky, unpublished data, January 1992). This exercise was designed to give them an idea of what supervision is and how to make it useful. It consists of having new trainees read a case example of a bad experience in supervision and then discussing what went wrong. Following that session, residents do a role play of a supervisory session in which the supervisor is giving feedback to the resident and the resident is trying to gain a better appreciation of the feedback given. This exercise also orients residents to practical facts about supervision ranging from how to videotape a session to how to take process notes. When polled, the residents unanimously found this type of formalized introduction to supervision quite useful as well as enjoyable. They reported feeling more empowered to approach supervision as informed consumers even before they had their first supervisory sessions.

From this exercise, it can be inferred that a supervisor who can engage in a similar exercise, even on an individual basis, will help make supervision more useful.

Similarly, Sadavoy and colleagues reported that "both (the beginning therapist and patient) are engaged in a difficult task for which only a minimal structure is provided, engendering much frustration, anxiety, misperception and a desire for guidance and reassurance" (Greben et al. 1973, p. 476) and recommended that a supervisory contract be established parallel to the therapeutic contract. In this way the "nonthreatening and respectful" supervisor referred to in the first section of this chapter can ameliorate the feelings of frustration and anxiety not just with his or her manner, but also by providing a frame or context for the supervision. Speaking about the uses and expectations of the supervision is very helpful, especially if it occurs before the patient has been seen. Allowing the resident to voice some of his or her own needs or wishes establishes from the beginning the necessary two-way flow of communication. Also, an invitation to speak freely about the supervisory process and the supervisor-supervisee relationship models for the resident the necessary reflection on the therapeutic process and the therapist-patient relationship. It also allows problem within the supervision to be addressed.

When first dealing with a psychotherapy patient, the resident frequently wishes for instruction and direction about highly pragmatic issues that he or she has never confronted before. Questions such as "how do you arrange the chairs?", "do you take notes?", "what do you say when a patient asks about your private life?", and "how do you confront someone about a missed appointment?" are examples of areas of ignorance and sources of anxiety for the novice therapist. At this stage, a supervisor who offers straightforward advice such as "you might consider saying . . . " is felt to be supportive, useful, and understanding of the resident's anxiety or indecision.

Later in training, however, a resident has evolved techniques for dealing with this kind of "frame" issue and frequently looks to the supervisor for a different kind of input. This is a move from requiring information to requiring ideas. The primary issue now is not how to respond but rather a more analytic (if not necessarily psychoanalytic) understanding of the sessions, including such issues as countertransference, parallel process, or metapsychology. One way of ensuring this mix is to have several supervisors throughout the training—each individual supervisor comes with his or her own expertise and experience, and therefore a combination of supervisors can enhance the residents' experience.

How both supervisor and supervisee act may be most influenced by the roles they see themselves in personally, within the academic setting. For the resident, the dual nature of being taught and judged simultaneously creates difficulty in making the supervision safe. Encouraging rapport or conveying a sense of safety may be encouraged by placing the supervisor outside the immediate context of academic achievement and grading. On the one hand, it is necessary for the supervisee to candidly reveal the sessions' contents and their own acts and affects to benefit from supervision. But this same material may be embarrassing or feel like a mistake, and the resident may be keenly aware of the fact that there is a power differential between him- or herself and the supervisor, who might be considered an evaluator more then a supervisor. It often seems that supervisors who are perceived as being "outside the system" of academic grading are also perceived as being safer in terms of self-disclosure. Rapport with these supervisors may therefore be more easily established.

Within a single training department where a core of faculty will have access to the evaluations, an element of "paranoia" is not an unusual defense for the supervisee. For this reason, it should be clear when establishing the contract that any feedback will be provided directly to the trainee first. If this is able to happen, inevitably the experience will be more useful for the trainee, as he or she will be able to discuss the feedback and process it within the context of the supervisory relationship. The anxiety of receiving direct, specific feedback can thus enhance learning rather than prevent it.

In some systems where the supervisor is absolved of direct clinical responsibility for the patient (usually by one psychiatric administrator being responsible for all such patients), the focus of the supervisor's role may then be absolutely on the education of the resident (see Figure 6–1). This can occur, without the problems of the patient "intruding," as it were, on the supervisory process. There are pros and cons to this approach. It encourages the resident's independence and responsibility for the patient as the supervisor is essentially unknown to the patient. It allows the use of process notes, which also give the resident freedom to focus the supervision on the issue of his or her choice rather than what the supervisor deems most interesting in a video- or audiotape. On the whole, it seems most suited to more senior residents—and perhaps to more psychoanalytically informed supervision, where the emphasis may legitimately be placed on the unconscious processes occurring within the patient and therapist, and the supervisee has sufficient clinical acumen to safeguard the patient's well-being.

A different role within a different system places a supervisor in a position of clinical responsibility for the patient. In such a case, the supervision is not linear but rather triangular (see Figure 6–2). Here it may be more usual to use audio- or videotaping of the sessions, or perhaps direct interviewing of the patient by the supervisor, as the material is more "accurately" presented (i.e., free of interpretation by the resident). Again, there are pros and cons. Residents (and patients), once their anxiety about observation has been reduced, often feel more supported in this model. If the supervisor is possessed of the tact and other qualities mentioned here, the supervisee will be able to benefit from input about posture, level of interest, and interpersonal style, and not only on his or her reported verbal interven-

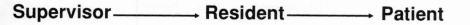

Supervisor ⟶ Resident ⟶ Patient

Figure 6–1. Linear supervision.

tions. The supervisor will also be guessing less about what the patient is like or how the therapist-patient interaction is going.

Being better informed should lead to more helpful suggestions about how to manage events within the therapy. It may even allow the crucial countertransference of the resident to be made explicit by tactful questioning about an observed stance or attitude of the resident that would have been unreported otherwise, precisely because it was a defensive and unconscious reaction. However, if this is not done with tact, the resident has no shield (as he or she does with process notes) and may feel threatened by the "overanalysis" of his or her way of being with the patient. On the other hand, a resident may be in this supervisory "triangle" earlier on in training and may find the direct, focused feedback more useful.

Perhaps the issue here is really one of flexibility. Some supervisors, residents, or situations will work best with videotape, whereas others may be best with process notes. The supervisor or system that can adapt to either in an empathic manner will allow the resident sufficient safety to communicate and learn easily in keeping with his or her individual stages of development.

It is worth noting that factors outside the immediate supervisor-supervisee relationship can have a positive impact upon it. Perez and colleagues (1984) noted that residents in programs that offered a core seminar in individual psychotherapy reported a more positive evaluation of their experience in supervision. Perez and colleagues hypothesized that this may be because of an increase in a resident's understanding of theoretical issues, thereby allowing them to more

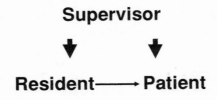

Figure 6–2. Triangular supervision.

actively participate in supervision. Perhaps it could also be that if a resident has other sources of psychotherapeutic knowledge, he or she has a greater tolerance for a supervisor who is less than optimal, as not all the resident's eggs are in one basket.

Granet and colleagues (1990) have suggested that junior supervisors face a variety of difficulties that may be reduced through formal education and training in supervision. In fact, several authors have described groups of various formats for the supervisors themselves. Kraft Goin and Klein (1974) noted that "as residents need experience, supervision, and instruction to be good therapists, therapists need experience, supervision, and instruction to become good supervisors" (p. 213). Morgan and colleagues (1984) reported on a group where one supervision was examined by a videotape, and Frayn (1991) reported on a psychotherapy supervision group that has evolved through several formats. Both authors have suggested means of improving such groups but agree they were beneficial to the participants. Frayn noted that "several supervisors began to mention that they found they were able to listen better and found it easier during supervision [after involvement in a supervisory group]" (p. 35). It seems likely that such approaches elevate the supervisory experience for the supervisee as well.

It is also the case that peer supervision eliminates many of the difficulties that can occur with a senior supervisor, and it therefore has a substantial role in a resident's psychotherapeutic education (E. Wallace, personal communication, January 1992). Peer supervision is, by definition, collegial, not formally open to grading, and often exquisitely attuned to this stage of training. These factors make it a safe and effective backstage in which to discuss issues. It is also a way that the formal supervision may be metabolized and put in context by comparing it with the experience of others. Potentially, it also serves as a means of disseminating or cross-pollinating various teachings, as a different resident may have dealt with the situation in his or her own supervision and can share that approach with a contemporary.

The establishment of rapport within other forms of psychotherapy may not be the same as in individual psychotherapy supervision. It seems that both group and family therapy are initially resisted by many residents, and the supervision is therefore often focused on getting started for some time. Perhaps these modalities exaggerate many of the issues discussed so far. For instance, early on in training, it may be uncertain how to deal with one patient who is seen privately; but it can be a matter of fear to deal with a room full of patients more publicly in a group. Similarly, a resident may be tentatively willing to reveal information about him- or herself in an individual psychotherapy supervision. To embark on a course (such as family therapy supervision) that could expose not just a resident but his or her family's own peculiar brand of craziness may be more threatening. For these reasons, supervisors in group and family work have to be especially attuned to the resident's situation to create a space where residents may discuss their work with intellectual and emotional freedom.

Good supervision, just like good therapy, requires clear boundaries. When a supervisor reacts in a therapist role with a supervisee as a patient, rather than as a teacher with a student, these boundaries may become blurred. Obviously, self-examination of actions, reactions, and affects provides the meat of the supervision, but it is important to avoid turning supervision into therapy. Residents who complain about supervisors not infrequently feel that the supervisors have made use of material to intrude in some way with an interpretation about *them* rather than deal with difficulties with patients. It is the direction of the interpretation rather than its content that is at fault.

No matter how accurate the "therapeutic" intervention may be, it demands an unsettling role shift for the resident from therapist to patient. The resident, especially if early in training or not in personal therapy, may be inclined to "clam up," and the supervision then loses its substance and impetus. Happily, learning can be therapeutic; but if the aim of supervision becomes therapy, it is unlikely to be educational. After all, the contract with the resident is an educational one. Without a psychotherapeutic contract, what Friedman (1981) describes as "therapeutic supervision" can "easily deteriorate into harassment when the supervisee needs comfort more than anything else" (p. 100). Ultimately, it seems that the most useful way for a supervisor to act with the resident is in a way that best promotes introspection on the part of the resident, which then allows him or her to respond more appropriately to the patient.

When the resident is not in individual therapy or analysis, the supervisor may become the main and perhaps exclusive model for the supervisee's therapeutic attitudes and behaviors. The rapport that is then established allows a kind of reversal of flow in the parallel process such that supervisory attitudes toward the trainee become reflected in a similar attitude of the trainee toward the patient. According to Friedman (1981), a "supervisor may recommend a therapeutic attitude but *demonstrate* an untherapeutic one" (p. 102). In such an instance it is undoubtedly more likely that the resident will learn the demonstrated rather than the recommended attitude. As the Markson report states, "the clinical attitude, which cannot be taught by instruction, should be exemplified by the supervisor's behavior as a teacher and an effective ally whenever problems arise in the supervisory relationship" (Greben et al. 1973, p. 477). Alternatively, "one shows how to take responsibility for providing help by providing help.".

Conclusion

It would seem that the greatest benefit of supervision, not surprisingly, occurs when the trainee is an active participant in his or her own learning and the supervisor is "good enough." This is the case when the supervisor is perceived as an expert colleague who can create a comfortable environment for supervision within which material can be conveyed in a manner that is attuned to the resident's individual needs. The attributes of a successful supervisory relationship such as genuineness, knowledge, and empathic understanding are crucial, not least of all because they are also the hallmarks of successful therapies.

References

Frayn DH: Supervising the supervisors: the evolution of a psychotherapy supervisors' group. Am J Psychother 45:31–42, 1991

Friedman L: A philosophy of psychotherapy supervision. Psychiatr Q 53:100–104, 1981

Gale MS: Resident perception of psychotherapy supervision. Compr Psychiatry 17:191–194, 1976

Granet MB, Kalman TP, Sacks MH: From supervisee to supervisor: an unexplored aspect of the psychiatrist's education. Am J Psychiatry 137:1443–1446, 1990

Greben SE, Markson ER, Sadavoy J: Resident and supervisor: an examination of their relationship. Canadian Psychiatric Association Journal 18:473–479, 1973

Kline F, Kraft Goin M, et al: You can be a better supervisor. Journal of Psychiatric Education 1:174–179, 1977

Kraft Goin M, Kline FM: Supervision observed. J Nerv Ment Dis 158:208–213, 1974

Miller CD, Oetting ER: Students react to supervision. Counsellor Education and Supervision 6:73–74, 1966

Morgan DW, Hamilton CS, Harris LH: Enhancing supervision of psychotherapy. South Med J 77:1406–1409, November 1984

Nelson GL: Psychotherapy supervision from the trainee's point of view: a survey of preferences. Professional Psychology 9:539–550, 1978

Pate LA, Wolff TK: Supervision: the resident's perspective. Academic Psychiatry 14:122–128, 1990

Perez EL, Krul LE, Kapoor R: The teaching of psychotherapy in Canadian psychiatric residency programs: residents' perceptions. Can J Psychiatry 29:658–664, 1984

Rice D, Fey W: Student satisfaction with small group teaching of psychiatry. Arch Gen Psychiatry 23:174–179, 1970

Shanfield SV, Gil D: Styles of psychotherapy supervision. Journal of Psychiatric Education 9:225–232, 1985

Chapter 7

Supervision of Group Psychotherapy

Molyn Leszcz, M.D., F.R.C.P.C., and
Leo Murphy, M.D., F.R.C.P.C.

Training in group psychother-
apy involves four main components: didactic learning, observation
of group therapy, experiential group participation, and supervision
of clinical work (Dies 1981; Lakin et al. 1969; Levin and Kanter
1964). Although all four elements are important, both from the perspective of the trainee (Kahn et al. 1986; Perez et al. 1984; Salvendy
et al. 1990) and that of the supervisor (Dies 1981), supervision is the
single most influential element within training, regardless of the theoretical model of group therapy employed. Group therapy training
is offered throughout psychiatry residency training programs in
North America (Pinney 1986), although the quality of supervision
requires further attention and improvement (Perez et al 1984).

In this chapter, we address group therapy supervision by examining the trainee's reactions to the unique aspects of group therapy,
the tasks of supervision and the supervisory relationship, and the
range of models of group therapy supervision.

The Trainee's Reactions to the Unique Aspects of Group Therapy

A dream reported in supervision by an inexperienced resident anticipating the start of his psychotherapy group is illuminating.

> I walked into the group therapy room. I was surprised to see 15 people present, all of whom were fellow residents, waiting for me to initiate group therapy with them. My former chief resident stood out as one individual I could identify in this crowd, and he was coming to me for treatment. I became very anxious, turned around and walked out.

Examination of this dream speaks to the intense anxiety trainees often experience when they begin to do group psychotherapy.

The experience of anxiety in response to difficult clinical situations, reflecting fears of loss of self-esteem and fears of ineffectiveness, is common in experienced psychotherapists conducting individual psychotherapy (Menninger 1990). It is all the more prevalent for beginning group therapists. Such anxiety is manifested commonly and with sufficient frequency that supervision should be prepared to address it from the very start of the supervisory process (Levin and Kanter 1964). Anxiety stems from many sources, reflecting unique aspects of group psychotherapy. Issues include fear of loss of control, fear of incompetence, fear of being overwhelmed by the sheer volume of material, fear of the group's disintegrating with premature terminations, and feelings of heightened personal and professional exposure, with the risk for subsequent shame and humiliation. A central concern is the uncertainty of dealing with group process, which contrasts with the more familiar and comfortable dyadic approach (Dies 1981).

Unlike in individual therapy, the group therapist will be exposed often to the scrutiny of a number of patients, the cotherapist, and (in some instances) observers who may be viewing his or her work from behind a one-way mirror. Feelings of shame and conflicts about exposure are particularly noxious. Not only do they inhibit the therapist in his or her clinical activity, but they also inhibit and diminish the trainee's willingness to discuss difficulties in supervision, hence perpetuating impediments to therapist development.

The anxiety stimulated by the therapist's engagement with the group in the face of the regressive pull of cascading emotions, and the potential diffusion of ego boundaries present in an unstructured psychotherapy group, coupled with the pressure a group can mount on an individual who wishes to be accepted and liked, combine to be enormously stressful (Saravay 1975; Yalom 1966). The therapist's defensive reactions and efforts at mastery have significant bearing on whether the group will survive and thrive. Williams (1966) has elaborated on the neophyte group therapist's fears and fantasies of group dyscontrol, disintegration, and the therapist's personal failure. He describes reactive stances ranging from withdrawal and avoidance of affect and engagement to obsessive control, gratification, and submission, with the consequent inability to set limits or establish effective group norms.

Initial, accurate interventions that may fall like the proverbial "lead balloon" producing no apparent useful group response can further delimit a therapist's range of therapeutic activity, as the neophyte underestimates the relative accuracy of his or her understanding in the face of the resistance of the group members. Hence, it is not surprising that unsupervised trainees become progressively less effective therapists over time. The absence of instruction about managing group members' resistances and group developmental difficulties reduces by attrition potentially effective therapist attributes that appear to the trainee to be of little use (Ebersole et al. 1969). Stein (1975) notes that even therapists who are quite experienced in individual therapy experience significant anxiety at the prospect of starting group psychotherapy. Unaided, the group therapist's development will fail to progress beyond the initial phases of feelings of shock and self-doubt (Zaslav 1988).

The therapist's primary tool is his or her use of self. In the group setting, a therapist is unable to avoid public exposure of how he or she uses this tool (Zinberg 1985). Prominent narcissistic issues and feelings of shame may emerge for the therapist when confronted with the gap between his or her current abilities and ideal professional sense of self (Alonso 1989). In psychodynamic group psycho-therapy, the therapist has important roles to fulfill as a facilitator of group interaction, and a participant and model, through his or her own therapeutic transparency and reactions to the individuals in the group and the group as a whole, in addition to traditional interpretive functions. The therapist is part of the social microcosm of the group and a recipient of interpersonal feedback. She cannot stay outside of the group process. Similarly, recognition of group developmental factors inherent in the development of group cohesion, as well as other unique group phenomena such as scapegoating, subgrouping, and dropouts from therapy, are additional factors the neophyte group therapist must encompass (Yalom 1966). The trainee is there-fore faced with an enormous range of stimuli and, because of his or her anxiety, a diminished and potentially diminishing range of effec-tive responses. A vicious cycle of either noisy or quiet disengagement in the group may ensue, resulting in the realization of the neophyte's greatest fear—group demoralization and disintegration.

> During a phase of group instability marked by the premature termination of its only two male members, a group consisted of five female members and a female group therapist. The manifest attitude of the group members became a giddy, self-denigrating one about their ability to be effective as a women-only group. In supervision, the group therapist responded that she felt inar-ticulate in the group meeting and quite constricted in her ability to intervene. However, it was apparent to her that the group members were anxious about the ability of the group to survive the loss of two male participants.
>
> In supervision, the trainee began to examine her own anxiety about being able to lead the group effectively. The group's self-denigration and demoralization made her feel devalued and de-moralized. Supervision served to detoxify this negative projection by examining the group process and its impact on the therapist, and promoting her responding to the group instability with a stronger statement of her own presence, eagerness, and ability to work effectively with the group. Some men might be added to the group to return its composition to a more natural balance. But the group would continue to function effectively,

and the current period would provide the women in the group with a special opportunity to look at their own attitudes of self-worth and self-devaluation in relationship to men.

Periods of group instability are particularly stressful times for trainees who lack the experience and associated confidence to be able to put into context group members' negative and self-devaluing comments, both about themselves and the therapeutic modality. The phenomenon of group instability is particularly prominent in the many training programs where neophyte trainees come into an ongoing group in the transition phase from the end of one academic year to the beginning of the next, replacing a group therapist who has terminated his or her involvement with the group (Long et al. 1988). Furthermore, in the absence of the therapist's understanding of interventions necessary for containment and holding, group cohesion will falter, and the group may indeed disintegrate (Hawkins 1986). Proactive supervision that can anticipate these particular difficulties and provide practical strategies for intervention is of the utmost importance in facilitating a successful initiation of training.

The Task of Supervision and the Supervisory Relationship

Because of these considerations, many authors think that the establishment of a satisfactory supervisor-supervisee relationship is essential (Dies 1981; Levin and Kanter 1964; Liebenberg 1981; Yalom 1985). Ideally, most begin before the actual initiation of the group and selection of patients. As important at the outset as didactic teaching of the theoretical background of group therapy is the opportunity to have the trainee's fears, anxieties, and apprehensions anticipated and modulated by the supervision process. How this develops is affected by the personalities of the supervisor and supervisee. But the preferred situation is one in which the supervisor sees him- or herself as a teacher, willing to share personal experiences about similar situations (both successes and failures) with a view to facilitating the development of the supervisee in a primary way.

The establishment of a learning alliance is a prerequisite (Alonso 1989). Important components of this alliance include principles of collaboration, mutual openness and respect, and reciprocity regarding the potential for both the supervisee and supervisor to learn from one another (Khan 1974). Accordingly, framing the trainee's learning of group psychotherapy along a developmental continuum may safeguard against a pathologizing process in which errors reflect personal or intractable professional deficits.

Our recent study of the experience of 16 neophyte group trainees in a large residency training program (L. Murphy, M. Leszcz, unpublished data, October 1992) concluded that although most trainees are satisfied and often view the group therapy experience as a highlight of their training, a significant number feel dissatisfied and plan to have nothing further to do with group psychotherapy. Although all trainees experience intense emotional reactions in the conduct of group psychotherapy, dissatisfied trainees reported a broader range of negative affects, including strong feelings of impotence, resentment, and hostility to their group. Complaints about technical difficulties alone did not distinguish satisfied from unsatisfied trainees; rather, the quality of the supervision experience was the chief variable associated with training satisfaction. Dissatisfied residents reported feeling "unheard," "criticized," and "talked to and unhelped," in contrast with satisfied residents who felt "supported" and "empathized with." These descriptors, emerging from open-ended interviews, are best summarized respectively by the comments of one trainee who claimed, "everything I did was wrong in the eyes of my supervisor," in contrast to the response of another who felt, "the supervisor made sense of my negative feelings."

Residents surveyed about their psychotherapy training in other studies (Pate and Wolff 1990; Perez et al. 1984) cite three critical elements in effective supervision: the supervisor's capacity for rapport with the supervisee, the supervisor's ability to identify supervisee psychotherapy shortcomings and help the supervisee overcome these, and the supervisor's ability to teach. Borrowing from Winnicott, Pate and Wolf (1990) comment that trainees seek a "good enough" supervisor—someone who encompasses technical expertise while developing a respectful collaborative relationship.

Attention paid to the supervisee-supervisor relationship is important and facilitates the objective of training, which is the transfer and acquisition of knowledge and competence. As the concepts of cohesion and therapeutic alliance are pivotal to the success of both group and individual therapy, so is the supervisor-supervisee relationship pivotal to the success of training. In the absence of trust, in order not to be unnecessarily devalued or diminished through the process of supervision, the trainee will likely direct his or her energy not to learning, but to the protection of his or her sense of self, and will devote energies to managing the supervision (Hutt et al. 1983) and to the avoidance of self-disclosure (see Chapter 13).

The central importance of the relationship with the supervisee does not preclude the supervisor's responsibility to the patients under the trainee's treatment. Excessive criticalness (Alonso 1989) will amplify the trainee's feeling of shame and relative incompetence, inhibiting his or her development as a therapist. Openness, support, opportunity for identification with the supervisor, and normalization of the therapist's anxieties will promote the therapist's development. Supervision should also promote the trainee's capacity to maintain a "space for thinking" (Mollon 1989), to retain therapeutic objectivity and perspective on the process of the treatment, and on his or her countertransference in the face of intense affects and projections from members of the group. It is from within this "space" that understanding and effective interventions emerge that feel like they belong to the therapist, rather than ones that feel co-opted from the supervisor.

The concept of isomorphy (Nicholas 1989), defined as the parallelism of structure and self-organizational processes among living systems, extends Ekstein and Wallerstein's (1958) concept of parallel process to a systemic view of the group-therapist-supervisor relationships, in which each contributor to the system has an impact on the others, and input at any level affects the others. The concept of parallel process—the dynamic linking of the process of psychotherapy to the process of supervision—by emphasizing the therapist's unconscious acting-out behavior in the supervision of difficulties experienced within the treatment relationship may have the inadvertent effect of stimulating the therapist's identification with the patient.

What he or she may actually require is further opportunity to identify with the supervisor, as the supervisee attempts to consolidate a professional self-identity.

The supervisor's willingness to explore and disclose personal reactions to the clinical material and the supervisory process, or his or her own previous experiences, models tolerance for not knowing all the answers, for risk taking, and for the emotional aliveness that the group leader requires to conduct effective group therapy. This can reduce the dread the trainee may feel about making an erroneous intervention, recognizing instead that the only serious mistake a therapist makes is to deny that he or she has made a mistake. In both supervision and therapy, transparency and disclosure must be in the interest of bolstering the supervision and the treatment, respectively, and not for the supervisor's or therapist's self-aggrandizement.

A male resident in supervision with the same supervisor for two different groups related that the two groups felt very different for him. The first group was one that he composed and began. In this group, he felt emotionally present, eagerly anticipating the sessions, and he thought that the degree of self-disclosure and interaction in the group was quite high. The second group was one that the resident took over at the beginning of the academic year. He felt much less interested in the second group, experiencing it as plodding and passive, and he viewed it as a necessary service requirement.

The reported emotional tone in the groups also was present in the two supervision hours, and the supervisor commented that he also noted that it seemed he had much more to contribute to the first group than to the second. The issues crystallized when a member of the second group complained to the therapist that he found the therapist to be very distant and unengaged in the group, as though he were putting in time. Although the patient was willing to consider that he often felt a hunger for greater emotional engagement, reflecting his feelings of emotional deprivation from having been in foster care during the early years of his youth, he added that he felt there was something real about his complaints to the therapist.

In exploration during supervision, the therapist in fact recognized that he felt like a "foster" therapist in this group, "filling in," unlike the first group, which he felt he conceived and constructed. This crystallization made immediate sense, and the supervisor added that he himself had wondered about such a dynamic. He had avoided raising it, however, because he himself had begun to believe that the continuing group was in fact an inferior one that had suffered from yearly transitions in therapists.

Following this discussion, the therapist was able to return to the group and begin to address in a realistic and respectful way the group member's complaints. He recognized that this group in particular required his full and total commitment, as it required each member's full and total commitment, to offset the impact of changeover in therapists. This was an issue that could be encompassed, rather than one that needed to be accepted as a discouraging reality.

The concept of choice point analysis (Tauber 1978) is instructive. It promotes a model of collaborative examination within supervision of clinical problems, and the range of interventions that are suitable, by studying the factors that contribute to each situation, attendant treatment options, and potential results. Developing the capacity to intervene at various levels of inference is an important therapeutic skill that trainees need to attain, to reduce their propensity to intervene in either one of two modes—to overstimulate the group, or to avoid an issue entirely because it feels too charged. Elucidation of a range of alternative approaches and interventions for the therapist reduces the propensity to use rigid, dyadic-based approaches to group psychotherapy (Yalom 1985) and may encourage using the here and now of the group in ways that are supportive rather than only confrontational.

In supervision of a long-term ego-supportive group for chronically impaired patients, the therapist reported that a recent group demonstrated in a clear fashion the way in which a particular group member contributed to his own isolation and loneliness (his chief complaints). While asking for feedback about what to do about his chronic sense of alienation, this patient ignored the feedback offered to him, considering it irrelevant. The therapist felt that he could not seize the opportunity to process what had just occurred, because he was certain that it would be hostile, hurtful, and damaging to the patient. The task of finding palatable ways of saying unpalatable things was examined in supervision in terms of the need to identify (in an empathic, nonattacking fashion) clear illustrations in the here and now of the group of what the patient did that bred his own loneliness. Surely other group members recognized this process and were also afraid to speak to it.

The therapist was encouraged to consider in the next such occurrence, starting at the lowest level of inference, by asking the particular patient what he was feeling at the time and asking for input, progressing as required to a higher level of inference about the patient's need perhaps to protect his sense of vulnerability by derogating people around him. Could it be that this is what was happening in the group at that time? Could he imagine how others felt on being told that their contribution was not worthwhile to him? Did he wish to push others away?

Issues related to countertransference are particularly complex ones in supervision. It is important to maintain the boundary between education and therapy. This is most challenging when the countertransference issue is in fact idiosyncratic to the therapist and truly a countertransference, rather than an understandable reaction to a difficult situation. It is difficult to enable the supervisee to identify and handle blocked areas in him- or herself while simultaneously retaining respect for personal privacy. Here too, the importance of the supervisor's being able to speak the unspeakable objectively, without being judgmental, provides a useful model for the trainee. The supervisor should not interpret but rather should only comment on what he or she observes. Exploration of the motivation of the therapist's reactions (in particular its genetic components), even if invited, is a boundary violation that may be deleterious.

A male therapist reported difficulty with an attractive woman in his group. She was quite striking both in appearance and in her very helpful and stimulating feedback in the group. She exercised a significant amount of power in the group; and although she was quite helpful to other members, she kept her own emotional life distant from the group. Fairly regularly, she would make teasing sexual comments to the therapist, complimenting him on his clothes. At one point, she commented to him in a session in which he was particularly active that the group "brought out the animal" in him.

Although he recognized the need to address this, the therapist felt apprehensive about inquiring about the patient's tendency to sexualize her relationship with him in the group, notwithstanding that this was a pattern in her external relationships. He was encouraged in supervision to synthesize the various remarks the patient made until he thought a suitable opportunity was present to address them. Protracted avoidance would no doubt impede the group's progress, as reflected by one member of the group raising his eyebrows knowingly, when the female patient made the comment about "bringing out the animal." The therapist believed his largest difficulty was that he felt embarrassed about potentially exposing his own attraction toward this patient.

In a subsequent group session, during which another patient made a sexual joke, this female patient talked about using sex as a way to maintain some form of closeness without becoming too emotionally intimate. When the therapist inquired whether that was what she was doing with him in the group, as he sometimes felt hesitant to approach her and examine more deeply what she was feeling, other members of the group supported him. This led to further exploration and clarification that in fact this patient's manifest sexualizing of issues in the group was defensive and warded off feelings of dependence and fears of disempowerment linked to sexual abuse early in her life. In her efforts to master these vulnerabilities, by turning the passive into the active, the patient had the potential to constrict and disempower the group and the therapist.

Models of Supervision

A variety of formats for supervision exist (Dies 1981; Liebenberg 1981; McGee 1968). These include a dyadic model in which one supervisor supervises a single group therapist, a dyadic model in which a more experienced group therapist coleads with and supervises a junior cotherapist, triadic supervision in which one supervisor supervises a cotherapy team, and group supervision in which a number of group therapists meet together. There are advantages and limitations to all models, and no research exists to argue for which model is superior. However, because it is often the group process that provides the beginning therapist with the greatest area of technical challenge (Dies 1981), supervision formats are enhanced when an opportunity exists to examine the process of multilateral relationships and interactions within the supervision (Lakin et al 1969), as well as the interpersonal processes and interpersonal style of the therapist.

Dyadic Supervision

Dyadic supervision provides an opportunity for relatively intensive exploration and detailed examination of the supervisee's experience in the group. The neophyte may also be afforded a substantial amount of support from the supervisor. However, Grossman and Karmiol (1973) have argued that this model may stimulate too narrow an identification on the therapist's part with the supervisor, and it may be harder to stimulate the therapist's own therapeutic style. Additionally, the supervision will suffer from limitations of reportage reflecting blind spots of the therapist's perceptions of the group (McGee 1968). A diminished opportunity to attend to interactive processes tends to emphasize dyadic, one-to-one models of therapy and may serve to perpetuate the primacy of the individual psychotherapy mode within the context of the group.

Cotherapy with dyadic supervision is an apprenticeship model in which a more experienced group therapist coleads with and supervises a trainee. Benefits of such a model include the trainee's opportunity to observe directly how an experienced therapist conducts group psychotherapy. Similarly, the junior therapist may be able to receive direct feedback from the supervising therapist about his or her therapeutic style and use of therapeutic interventions. This can facilitate risk taking if the neophyte is comfortable with the senior therapist's support and availability to him or her. The presence of the coleader-supervisor enhances the trainee's fuller understanding of the group dynamics, because there is a reduction in potential blind spots.

This model works best when there is a realistic expectation between the coleaders that the junior leader can assume reasonable therapeutic responsibility (Yalom 1985). Coleadership is in fact exactly that. It is not a model of president and copresident; instead, both leaders are coleading. Without this understanding, the junior therapist is likely to feel stifled. The junior therapist may feel that he or she need not nor will ever obtain therapeutic ownership of the group. Group members may recognize that and role-lock the junior therapist into a position of relative ineffectiveness (Berman 1975). In this situation, the junior therapist may become a receptacle for projections from group members and displacements from the transference to the senior therapist. As in all models of cotherapy, issues of power, authority, dependence, and competitiveness must be addressed (Davis and Lohr 1971; McGee 1974).

> A beginning group therapist welcomed the opportunity of coleading a group with an experienced and well-respected group therapist. After 2 months, the new therapist still felt peripheral to the group and believed his contributions were ignored entirely by the group members. Despite support on the part of the senior group therapist, the junior therapist thought himself to be quite marginal in the group. In frustration, he commented that the group seemed locked into ignoring him and deferring to the more experienced, "wizened" group therapist in a way that struck him as reflecting passivity and unwillingness to take responsibility for themselves.
>
> This component of the intervention was in fact quite helpful to the group, by stimulating exploration of the group members' dependence on the senior therapist. What provided for even more interesting and humorous exploration in supervision was the neophyte therapist's overlooked parapraxis—using "wizened" instead of "wise"—reflecting the junior therapist's competitive and rivalrous feelings toward his more experienced colleague.

Triadic Supervision

The triadic supervision model, involving supervision of a cotherapy team by a supervisor, is a common vehicle for training (Davis and Lohr 1971; McGee 1968; McGee and Schuman 1971). It provides comprehensive reporting of the group in supervision, as the two therapists serve to correct each other's blind spots and different foci. Their ability to give one another feedback and together examine the group process, transference, and countertransferential developments within the group and the interpersonal processes can provide significant amounts of support and information. However, the cotherapy team is subject to its own process and dynamics, and supervision needs to address issues that invariably arise, including issues of competitiveness, dependency, and rivalry. How the cotherapy goes influences dramatically how the group will function. Hence, the cotherapy can be experienced as mutually supportive to the cotherapists, or conversely, can serve as a serious impediment (McGee and Schuman 1971). These issues emerge with such regularity that it is useful for the supervisor to identify their potential at the beginning of supervision and establish a contract with the cotherapy team to examine their relationship.

> An inexperienced psychiatric resident was paired with an experienced nonmedical female therapist in a psychotherapy group. Despite his lack of experience in group therapy and his apparent anxiety about participation as a group leader, he believed that he should be as active and intervening as his more experienced coleader. It quickly became apparent that his competitiveness with her, fueled in part by interdisciplinary and gender rivalry, led him to intervene in ways that were aimed at demonstrating his knowledge and prowess to the group, often contradicting his coleader. Instead of deepening her interventions when the group seemed resistant to them, he would invariably take the group off into a different and less useful direction.
>
> The process of supervision was difficult, as the resident was hostile and unable to acknowledge any limitations in his understanding of the group or the presence of conflict in the cotherapy. The phenomenon of working at cross purposes,

which was manifested in the group, was also manifested in supervision. Within 12 sessions, the resident decided not to continue in the psychotherapy group. After his withdrawal from the
group, his cotherapist reported a dream in which she felt she
was playing hockey and was her team's goalie. But a member
of her own team kept shooting the puck at her, and she wondered why this person was on her team.

Poorly allied or disengaged cotherapists will model for their
groups passivity and the inability to work through difficulties. This
inability may also serve as a nidus for patients' splitting and projection, especially when fertile ground for the growth of these projections exists within the relationship of the cotherapists around issues
of competitiveness, self-esteem, dependency, power, or the wish to
be the preferred or more effective coleader.

Supervision ideally encourages the development of an effective
relationship between the coleaders without siding with one or another in any conflict. A systemic view of the contributions of the
group, the cotherapy team, the supervision, and the multiple levels
of relationships both empowers the supervision and illuminates the
impact of interpersonal and group processes—an essential learning
component in group therapy. The supervisor similarly must limit
him- or herself to commenting only about observable phenomena,
rather than interpreting motivation. Whenever possible, linking the
cotherapy process to the group process may help resolve difficulties
between the cotherapists, as the only real supervisory leverage present is what is in the best interest of the treatment.

Supervision Group

This model of supervision consists of regular meetings of group therapists with a supervisor (Dies 1981; Liebenberg 1981). This model
most directly realizes group process and provides participants with
firsthand exposure to group dynamics through actual group participation. However, it is not intended to be a substitute for the experiential aspects of training in group psychotherapy. Additionally,
Sadock and Kaplan (1971) caution against turning the supervision
group into a form of "pseudogroup psychotherapy." A well-func-

tioning supervision group provides opportunities for support and learning from one another's difficulties and successes in ways that normalize the developmental process of the therapist's functioning. Furthermore, it offsets the potential bias of exposure to a single supervisor. However, there are numerous limitations with this model, in particular for neophyte trainees who may experience exacerbation of anxiety and self-doubt through their participation in a group. As such, it may be a useful adjunct, but it should probably not be the only format of supervision for beginning therapists. Additional difficulties arise when the participants in the group are at different levels of experience, or if they have prior relationships with one another that color their involvement in the group.

Liebenberg (1981) emphasizes the importance of the group's being essentially an opportunity to learn about a set of principles and techniques for the practice of group psychotherapy, rather than for primary illumination of the interpersonal style of the supervisees. The presentation of individual members and how they come across will influence the degree to which they can be identified and empathized with by their colleagues. However, this form of supervision requires a strong sense of cohesion and alliance between the participants and must be esteem enhancing. Participation in such a group does carry with it a potential for negative exposure and resultant feelings of shame or humiliation. A systemic view is best employed in this context as well. Such an approach looks at the contributions made to the supervision group process from the supervised treatments, the therapists or cotherapists, and the supervisor in addition to the process of the supervision group. Milieu or institutional factors may also need to be considered. Shifting from examination of the group's process to the level of content and didactic learning about group process provides an effective balance between the stimulation of supervisee affect and the ultimate goal of learning about technique and practice.

Cooper and Gustafson (1985) emphasize this format of supervision as a unique opportunity for the illumination and restructuring of individual therapists' fundamental unconscious paradigms about relationships. Working at its best, the supervision group functions as a form of transitional object (Schneider and Berman 1991), aiding the trainee in the move from comfortable and familiar paradigms to newer, more open ones, as he or she acquires new skills and consolidates a professional identity.

The supervisor must recognize a personal wish to treat and not submit to it, as his or her mandate is the trainee's performance in therapy and not his or her personhood. This requires clear boundaries about self-disclosure, and a clear set of expectations that material illuminated in the supervision group will be used to reflect processes within the conduct of group psychotherapy. Utilization of parallel process within the supervision group (in particular around issues of therapists' demoralization, dependence, and authority conflicts) is readily achieved through this model. The supervisor must be willing to demonstrate his or her own ability to shift from traditional paradigms regarding authority, dependence, and passivity, without abandoning the supervisory and teaching function. Cooper and Gustafson (1985) use the supervision group in a model similar to Balint's (1957) description of groups he conducted for general practitioners. The group should be guided by the principle of encouraging participants to develop the courage to examine their own limitations and ignorance, exposing actual therapeutic behavior, and in so doing illuminating habitual therapeutic errors.

Observation

In contrast with individual therapy, the group therapy trainee also has the opportunity of having his or her work observed directly by the supervisor. Through direct observation, supervision becomes potentially a live process, undiluted by anonymity and process notes. Vast differences can exist between the subjective report of the inexperienced group leader and the more objective perspective of an experienced supervisor, reducing blind spots in the supervisee-patient relationship. However, observation should not substitute for process notes or for the therapist himself conceptualizing and organizing the group session for presentation and supervision.

Mackie and Wood (1968) noted that the process of observation carries with it its own dynamics. Zinberg (1985) addressed similar issues in his elaboration of the difference between the private and public psychiatric interview. Observation ideally is experienced as a component of a mutual, collaborative, and collegial training relationship rather than as a fault-finding mission. Dies (1981) cites potential difficulties with observation, in terms of inhibition of the therapist (who fears failing and having this publicly scrutinized) as the protective myth of his or her therapeutic effectiveness may be dismantled by having the work scrutinized closely. An additional hazard is the risk of the therapist having his or her interventions aimed at obtaining approval from the supervisor, or being stimulated exhibitionistically, as exemplified by the trainee who listens eagerly to hear sounds from the viewing room indicating that the supervisor is there. Observation may in fact fuel learning resistances if the therapist feels observation is intended to be critical, competitive, or invariably seeking to take the side of the patient against the therapist (Mackie and Wood 1968).

In the context of a stable supervisory relationship, observation enhances the process of supervision, as the therapist's actual style in therapy can be observed firsthand, thereby reducing blind spots. Therapists may fail to report areas of difficulty or embarrassment (see Chapter 13). As important, however, is the fact that trainees often fail to identify effective interventions performed inadvertently; or conversely, they fail to capitalize fully on particularly rich moments in the group. Having a supervisor observe and later provide feedback to the trainee provides a useful vehicle for the linking of theory to effective clinical interventions. The process of observation may be further detoxified for the supervisee, through the supervisor having his or her own work open to observation by the trainees, thereby balancing the degree of exposure between them.

Conclusion

Regardless of the model of supervision employed, the objectives in terms of provision of technical information regarding group psychotherapy are the same. Without the leader's facilitation, structure, and appropriate intervention, it is unlikely that the psychotherapy group will become cohesive, and it is likely that the group will fragment and individual members will regress and drop out. As the trainee understands the concept of working with the group process, as opposed to focusing on individuals only; as he or she understands working with the here and now rather than focusing on reports of external events; and as he or she develops the ability to respond to group pressure and the role of group development, the trainee's capacity to facilitate is strengthened. The interactive nature of the group requires a much greater willingness on the part of its members to participate and to be exposed than does individual psychotherapy. The resistances that individuals will present to this engagement in the here and now become primary foci of the therapist's intervention (Yalom 1985).

As this process begins to mobilize, the therapist is able to see that he or she is not engaged in the process of treating the group, while feeling at risk of the group turning on its leader. Rather, he or she is working with the group, using its resources to treat its individual members. What appears initially as an overwhelming amount of information becomes more manageable as the therapist is able, through the aid of supervision, to place it in context and see it as linked to the group's psychological life and the members' internal worlds, rather than as a series of apparently disconnected and confusing pieces of information.

The enabling relationship between supervisor and supervisee should be a dynamic and reciprocal one in which both benefit and are able to teach one another (Liebenberg 1981). Boundaries between supervisor and supervisee are essential. But if a framework is maintained showing supervision to be an open, collaborative transaction, aimed at facilitating the professional development of the trainee, the work generally unfolds positively.

References

Alonso A: Shame and guilt in psychotherapy supervision. Paper presented at Mount Sinai Hospital Academic Day VIII, November 10, 1989

Balint M: Method and technique in the teaching of medical psychology. Br J Med Psychol 27:37–41, 1957

Berman AL: Group psychotherapy training. Small Group Behavior 6:325–344, 1975

Cooper L, Gustafson JP: Supervision in a group: an application of group theory. Clinical Supervisor 3:7–25, 1985

Davis FB, Lohr NE: Special problems with the use of co-therapies in group psychotherapy. Int J Group Psychother 7:143–158, 1971

Dies RR: Group psychotherapy: training and supervision, in Psychotherapy Supervision. Edited by Hess AK. New York, Wiley, 1981, pp 337–366

Ebersole GD, Leiderman H, Yalom ID: Training the nonprofessional group therapist. J Nerv Ment Dis 179:294–302, 1969

Ekstein R, Wallerstein RS (eds): The Teaching and Learning of Psychotherapy. New York, Basic Books, 1958

Grossman WK, Karmiol E: Group psychotherapy supervision and its effect on resident training. Am J Psychiatry 130:920–921, 1973

Hawkins DM: Understanding reactions to group instability in psychotherapy groups. Int J Group Psychother 36:241–260, 1986

Hutt CH, Scott J, King M: A phenomenological study of supervisees' positive and negative experiences in supervision. Psychotherapy: Theory, Research and Practice 20:118–123, 1983

Kahn EM, White EM, Hawkins DM: Training in group psychotherapy: residency experience, use in practise and self perception of competency. Journal of Psychiatric Education 10:204–211, 1986

Khan MMR: The Privacy of the Self. New York, International Universities Press, 1974

Lakin M, Lieberman MA, Whitaker DS: Issues in the training of group psychotherapists. Int J Group Psychother 19:307–325, 1969

Levin S, Kanter SS: Some general considerations in the supervision of beginning group psychotherapists. Int J Group Psychother 14:318–331, 1964

Liebenberg B: Multiple levels in psychoanalytically oriented group supervision. Int J Group Psychother 31:429–441, 1981

Long K, Pendleton L, Winter B: Effects of therapist termination on group process. Int J Group Psychother 38:211–222, 1988

Mackie R, Wood J: Observations on two sides of a one-way screen. Int J Group Psychother 16:117–185, 1968

McGee TF: Supervision in group psychotherapy: a comparison of four approaches. Int J Group Psychother 18:165–176, 1968

McGee TF: The triadic approach to supervision in group psychotherapy. Int J Group Psychother 24:471–470, 1974

McGee TF, Schuman BN: The nature of the co-therapy relationship. Int J Group Psychother 21:25–35, 1971

Menninger WW: Anxiety in the psychotherapist. Bull Menninger Clin 54:232–246, 1990

Mollon P: Anxiety, supervision and a space for thinking: some narcissistic perils for clinical psychologists in learning psychotherapy. Br J Med Psychol 62:112–113, 1989

Nicholas MW: A systemic perspective of group therapy supervision: use of energy in the supervisor-therapist-group system, in Variations on Teaching and Supervising Group Therapy. Edited by Lewis KG. New York, Haworth, 1989, pp 27–39

Pate LA, Wolff TK: Supervision: the residents' perspective. Academic Psychiatry 14:122–128, 1990

Perez EL, Krul LE, Kapoor R: The teaching of psychotherapy in Canadian psychiatric residency programs: residents' perceptions. Can J Psychiatry 29:658–663, 1984

Pinney EL: Group psychotherapy training in psychiatric residencies. Journal of Psychiatric Education 10:106–112, 1986

Sadock BJ, Kaplan HI: Training and standards in group psychotherapy, in Comprehensive Group Psychotherapy. Edited by Kaplan HI, Sadock BJ. Baltimore, MD, Williams & Wilkins, 1971

Salvendy JT, Robson B, Babiak T: Group psychotherapy in psychiatric residency training. Academic Psychiatry 14:27–33, 1990

Saravay SM: Group psychology and the structural theory: a revised psychoanalytic model of group psychology. J Am Psychoanal Assoc 23:69–89, 1975

Schneider S, Berman M: The supervision group as a transitional object. Group Analysis 24:65–72, 1991

Stein A: The training of the group psychotherapist, in Group Psychotherapy and Group Function. Edited by Rosenbaum M, Berger MM. New York, Basic Books, 1975, pp 684–704

Tauber LE: Choice point analysis—formulation, strategy, intervention and result in group process therapy and supervision. Int J Group Psychother 28:163–184, 1978

Williams M: Limitations, fantasies and security operations of beginning group therapists. Int J Group Psychother 16:152–162, 1966

Yalom ID: Problems of neophyte group therapists. Int J Soc Psychiatry 12:52–59, 1966

Yalom ID: The Theory and Practice of Group Psychotherapy, 3rd Edition. New York, Basic Books, 1985

Zaslav M: A model of group therapist development. Int J Group Psychother 38:511–519, 1988

Zinberg NE: The private versus the public psychiatric interview. Am J Psychiatry 142:889–894, 1985

Chapter 8

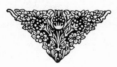

Family Therapy Supervision

Leopoldo Chagoya, M.D., F.R.C.P.C., and
Kenneth Citron, M.D., F.R.C.P.C.

T he evolving field of family psy-
chotherapy presents the clinician with new techniques with which to
treat interpersonal conflicts. Supervision varies accordingly to fit the
approach the supervisor teaches. As we note in Chapter 12, the supervisor conveys in his or her technique of supervising a philosophy
of therapy, a belief system about the causes and solutions of problems, and a template about how humans and relationships develop.
This philosophy (whether conscious or unconscious on the part of
the supervisor), combined with the bias determined by the school of
therapy being taught, results in different styles of supervision as part
of family therapy training (McDaniel et al. 1983).

For instance, the type of supervision necessary to teach White's
(1986) technique of externalizing the causes of conflicts is different
from the supervision necessary to teach De Shazer and colleagues'
(1986) Solution Focused Therapy. If supervisors wish to teach the
principles and technique of object relations family therapy (Scharff

We gratefully acknowledge the suggestions and ideas of Charlotte Chagoya, R.N., PG
Psych. Nurs., Dip.Fam.Ther., in the writing of this chapter.

and Savege Scharff 1987), they will supervise differently from the way they would if their objective were to train their students in the intricacies of feminist family therapy (Wheeler et al. 1989).

In the *Handbook of Family Therapy Training and Supervision* (Liddle et al. 1988), seven types of teaching are described for seven types of family therapy. These include structural therapy, the Milan approach, Bowenian therapy, the brief therapy model of Fisch and colleagues, the strategic or indirect techniques, the integrative psychodynamic and systems approach, and Haas and Alexander's functional family therapy. Each method is dealt with in a special chapter, with a description of what form of supervision is necessary to help the student develop within each theoretical framework.

Our comments in this chapter, of course, are necessarily bound by a theoretical bias. They involve an integrative approach. We have a basic psychoanalytic orientation, and we include in our teaching elements of systems, communication, and structural theories (Chagoya 1980, 1983). Our students are usually psychiatric residents rotating through a psychiatric service offering family therapy training (Mount Sinai Hospital in Toronto). The goal of the 1-year teaching is to whet the residents' appetite for the technique and the theory of dealing with family conflicts.

Whitaker and Keith (1981) distinguished three levels of training within the specialty:

1. Learning about family therapy (accomplished by attending a few weekend workshops with experts in the field);
2. Learning to do family therapy (accomplished by participating in seminars and supervision as part of a global training in another specialty); and
3. Becoming a family therapist (achieved by participating in a 2- or 3-year intensive training dedicated entirely to the theory, technique, and vicissitudes of family therapy).

In this chapter, we refer to the second level of teaching.

Because we, the authors, also function as individual psychotherapy supervisors for other residents, we pay special attention to the difference in the teaching when we are wearing the family therapy hat. As in any supervision, we scrutinize the therapist-supervisor relationship with a systems approach.

Systems theory (Bertalanffy 1968) and communication theory (Watzlawick et al. 1967) are part of the basis of all modes of family therapy. In the recent literature, however, it is as if the contribution of these theories were a given, and modern authors do not acknowledge it. Central to any family therapy training program is an understanding of systems and communication theories, as well as the knowledge of the family life cycle as described by McGoldrick and Carter (1982), so the student may establish the parallel between family stages and the psychosocial stages or "ages" Erikson (1968) described in the individual.

The term "isomorphism" designates the tendency of the relationship between trainer and trainee to mimic that of therapist and patient. It has also been designated "parallel process." The context of family therapy training is ideal for examining ideas of isomorphism between therapy and supervision, cross-cultural issues, and matters of power hierarchies, especially as they relate to racial discrimination and sex role stereotyping.

Family therapy supervision with psychiatric residents provides unique opportunities for different approaches to the therapist-supervisor teaching relationship. In individual psychotherapy supervision, confidentiality concerns have tended to limit the teaching to reviewing process notes that the therapist takes during or after the session. In family therapy supervision, a variety of modalities can be used to teach the therapist directly. Whiffen and Byng-Hall (1982) have published a perceptive analysis of these techniques. In addition to process notes, the supervisor may request an audiotape or a videotape of the therapy sessions (Bodin 1969) or organize "live" supervision with the resident (Berger and Dammann 1982).

When only process notes are used by the supervisee, the teacher can assess how much attention the student gives to the interaction, the amount of detail he or she can recall, and the countertransferential tone in which the session is told. The nonverbal communication of the resident is the key factor here. The disadvantage of the method is that the student may avoid, through obsessively written details, exposure of his or her technical difficulties or denied affect. Nevertheless, the supervisor can elicit (through tactful questions) the material absent from the notes.

When an audiotape is used, it is mandatory to insist on high-quality recordings so as not to strain the participants in trying to guess what a family member or the therapist said. The audiotape permits a clearer presentation of the sequence and the emotional tone of family interchanges. But it has a disadvantage. It is generally impossible to listen to a full session in one supervisory hour; the student can only have supervision of a portion of it. According to the level of trust the supervisee has in his teacher, he or she may select the best (to show his or her prowess) or the worst (to examine his or her deficiencies). A combination of verbal accounts and audiotapes of the sessions is effective.

When videotapes are used, it is similarly essential to have image and sound of decent quality. The videotape permits the most accurate review of the therapeutic experience, but it is time consuming and requires equipment and, at times, a technician (not always available in every teaching institution). It helps greatly if the person who handles the camera and decides what to film is somewhat in tune with what interests the therapist or the supervisor. A common mistake in video recording for supervision is to film only images of the family, never providing a full view of the therapist. Yet the trainee who watches him- or herself in action may learn a great deal about how he or she uses nonverbal communication as an advantage or as a hindrance in his or her style of interviewing.

When "live" supervision is the mode chosen (Berger and Dammann 1982), the supervisor may sit in the room with the student-therapist and act as a cotherapist; or he or she may act only as a commentator on the session process, as a consultant, speaking exclusively to the trainee. In this latter technique, at times the family tend to talk to the supervisor, ignoring their therapist. If this occurs, the supervisor has to be skillful in discouraging such a process. Also, therapist and supervisor should be comfortable about having a supervisory discussion in the presence of the family.

The supervisor must be careful not to take over the session. Even if he or she probably cannot help but radiate more confidence and experience in front of the family than the trainee, the supervisor must not unwittingly displace the inexperienced therapist. If he or she does, the supervisor will leave the supervisee with the difficult task of coping, after the consultation, with an idealized image the family may construct based on the brief contact with the supervisor. The idealization of the supervisor carries with it the devaluation of the student-therapist and consequent splitting.

"Live" supervision may be carried out from behind a one-way mirror. Andolfi and Menghi (1980), Cornwell and Pearson (1981), and Gershenson and Cohen (1978) have examined variations and vicissitudes in supervising family therapy this way. Behind the mirror, the supervisor may act alone or share the supervisory process with a group, the so-called "Greek chorus." The supervisor may observe only, leaving the therapist to his or her own devices, and after the session may comment on the content and process he or she has observed. Usually, however, the supervisor communicates with the trainee, either by phoning in messages or through the use of a small earphone or "bug in the ear." Phone calls are timed strategically to aid in the therapy, while the earphone provides the possibility of communicating more frequently with the supervisee, without the family necessarily being aware that this is occurring.

There is an amusing anecdote, however, about an instance when a family heard the message from the earphone before the therapist could understand it: they started explaining to the therapist what the supervisor had suggested! If neither the phone nor the earpiece is used, the trainee may have the freedom to interrupt the session with the family and go behind the mirror to consult with the observer or observers, who may suggest strategies or tasks for the family and the therapist. Because the family is always told about the presence of observers, they may relay messages to the family in writing or in person as part of the therapeutic-supervisory experience. Another possibility, when the student is stuck in a troublesome situation with the family, is for the supervisor to call the therapist out for a breather and to receive advice on how to extricate him- or herself from the difficulty. Finally, another variable is a preprogrammed break in the family session, where at a designated time the therapist will interrupt the therapy and go behind the mirror to exchange comments with the supervisor.

"Live" supervision has several advantages. It provides a direct observation of the student-family interaction and allows the immediate remediation of mistakes. It also offers peer consultation, strategic planning, didactic explanations, and support on the spot for the beginning therapist. Also, when the supervisor intervenes, it provides a living model of technique and attitude for the student. The supervisor teaches by showing how, not just by talking.

On the downside, during "live" supervision the interviewer has to cope with persecutory feelings that may paralyze him or her. The self-conscious supervisee may be too preoccupied with how he or she looks to the supervisor. This may distract the student, who might pay less attention to the family interaction and to the formulation of the interpersonal dynamics. An integrated view of the entire process may be delayed until this self-consciousness is overcome. Sources of performance anxiety for the supervisee include the family, the audience behind the mirror, and the video camera (when the session is being filmed while it is being observed). In addition, the supervisee may have to recall (during the session, while he or she interviews) some theoretical tenets, or struggle with countertransference issues stemming from his or her own family. Trust between the interviewer and the observing supervisor is of utmost importance. When there are several observers, the supervisor has to keep control of the quality of the exercise and prevent it from becoming a showing-off of brinksmanship, or a barrage of critical voices that may overwhelm the student. Finally, "live" supervision may be consultative and can be used occasionally rather than continuously, when problems in the therapy warrant it.

The material requirements for good "live" supervision are an adequate Gesell chamber with a wide one-way mirror; good-quality sound to perceive the voices of patients and therapists; and some administrative work to coordinate the time of the family, the therapist, the supervisor, and the peer group.

We believe that, whenever possible, it is preferable to supervise family therapy in small groups of three or four students. Such a context provides them with the experience of being seen, gets them used to peer pressure, gives them the opportunity to learn from others, allows them to function at times as supervisors of their colleagues, and teaches them to accept peer supervision and support. A supervision group may be multidisciplinary; for instance, it may include a psychiatric resident, a social work student, a psychoanalyst who wishes to learn family therapy, a psychology student, or a psychiatric nurse.

If a supervisory group is available, a good method of "live" supervision is the use of simulation or role-playing (Mansfield 1991). The student may portray him- or herself while other trainees playact the members of the supervised family. Or the student assumes the role of a family member with whom he or she is having difficulty, while a colleague or the supervisor plays the therapist. Role-playing can be used to supervise technique, by reproducing in the supervisory hour the obstacles and the impasses that the student gets into. Simulation can also be used to illustrate and make the student aware of how his or her own emotional reactions to the family can get in the way of becoming an effective therapist. Techniques, empathy, and countertransference cease to be theoretical when they are enacted in a simulation; the exercise becomes an experiential form of learning. Another useful aspect of simulation is that it desensitizes the student to being exposed. Family therapy is a form of treatment in which the therapist is constantly subjected to the scrutiny of family members. If the student gets used to being on display, he or she will experience less stage fright when facing different types of families (Burdill 1976).

Family therapy deals with systems, whereas individual psychotherapy focuses on the intrapsychic workings of the person, at times ignoring that we all are an integral part of a system. Any training in family therapy necessarily includes a reorientation toward systemic thinking, especially for students who have been indoctrinated into focusing only on the individual psyche as an isolated entity. If the student-therapist arrives at the family program with a preconceived approach based on individual psychodynamics, the transition to systemic thinking may be problematic and needs to be carefully nurtured by the supervisor. Through the use of literature and concepts that combine individual and systemic models (Nichols 1987; Steinhauer et al. 1984), student therapists can preserve their individual psychodynamic approaches without experiencing a loss, when they have to think in systemic terms. With the help of the supervisor, the trainee can gradually integrate individual and interpersonal system concepts to understand how families deal with their life together and with the outside world.

At times, to try a new approach, suspension of what has previously been learned is necessary. The success of this process largely depends on the strength of the supervisor/therapist relationship and on the therapist's capacity to trust and believe in the supervisor's methods and ability.

In any relationship, the fit of personalities determines the success of the venture. Problems may arise between therapist and supervisor when the latter teaches techniques that may be indirect, risky, and foreign to the student. If the therapist cannot see how these techniques will be useful, he or she may rebel against them either overtly or silently.

As in other forms of supervision, isomorphism must be watched for during family therapy teaching. Much like countertransference issues in individual supervision, it is not always wise to comment on the isomorphism. Nevertheless, the supervisor has to recognize it and work around it in the interest of the family's progress as well as that of the supervisee.

The supervisor must distinguish transference/countertransference phenomena from other matters between him or her and the therapist, and from issues stemming from the isomorphism between the therapy and the supervision. If the supervisor acts out a conflict toward the therapist, quite likely he or she will replicate such acting out toward the family.

A positive attitude in the supervisee includes trust and openness in presenting the family material, acceptance and use of the critical comments made by the supervisor or by peers, a healthy questioning of supervision recommendations, and, eventually, a creative adaptation of the supervisor's style of doing therapy.

A negative attitude in the supervisee may include antagonism or excessive skepticism toward the family method, self-fulfilling prophecies to prove the supervisor wrong, distrust and distortion in the session presentations, aggressive competition with peers, inability to use constructive critiques, a passive compliance with the supervisor's recommendation without self-elaboration, or triangulation wherein the student "consults" with other supervisors about the recommendations of the family therapy supervisor. In such instances, the student tends to adopt a persecuted stance.

When residents work only with inpatients in a psychiatric ward, they will limit their experience to the families that can visit such a setting. If the supervisor is not involved in the tensions and dilemmas the ward staff face, the possibility of splitting exists. This is especially problematic if the supervisor/therapist dyad is seen as treading on the territory of other professionals who are traditionally entrusted with the role of treating the family. In these circumstances, the supervisor has to supervise the resident, not only on his or her dealings with the family, but also on his or her dealings with the entire ward team system and its own interpersonal dynamics. Luckily, this proves to be good material for the family systems theory mill.

The usual resistances of supervisees toward delving into family therapy include a tendency to see family members in terms of stereotypical "bad guys" and "good guys"; a reluctance to contravene social graces through making interventions and directing sessions; an avoidance of crisis during the sessions; a premature search for recipes and solutions before understanding the complexities of an interaction problem; the use of cotherapy to hide behind a more experienced colleague; and the apparent impossibility to find a suitable family to start practicing the craft (Chagoya 1975).

From the point of view of the trainee, there tend to be four areas of focus in family therapy supervision: evaluative, internal, interactive, and "big picture" foci (Schwartz 1988). The evaluative focus deals with the trainee's need for approval from the supervisor. The internal focus concerns the trainees with their own behavior toward the family, either on audio- or videotape or in "live" supervision. The interactive focus considers the interpersonal family dynamics, and the "big picture" focus allows the supervisee to formulate problems and plan the treatment. Trainees need to be reassured in the area of evaluation to reduce their internal preoccupation. This way they can get on with the task of focusing on the family's interactions and the big picture. A balance between self-awareness and awareness of the family, with reference to and revision of the problem formulation, is ideal in ongoing family therapy training.

In the phrase "I do family therapy" we can summarize what a supervisor can offer a student through supervision.

- "I": The supervisee has to gradually realize who he or she is as a product of his or her own family, with prejudices, stereotypes of family functioning, and ethical, social, cultural, and moral values, which will influence his or her countertransference in the face of family conflicts.
- "Do": What is it that a family therapist is supposed to do in front of a family to help them reconceptualize their role in each problem? The student has to differentiate between counseling, educating, supporting, stimulating, questioning, challenging, confronting, prescribing assignments, interpreting, asking provocative or therapeutic questions, or waiting silently for an insight to take place or for the family to be ready to undertake a change-provoking task.
- "Family": The student has to accept that the nuclear traditional family is only one of many systems he or she will face as a unit of treatment. He or she may treat divorcing or divorced couples with children, homosexual couples with adopted children, homosexual couples raising the children of the previous marriage of one of the partners, bisexual parents with children, binuclear families with two sets of children from the previous marriage of each spouse as well as children of the remarried couple, families formed by individuals who live together or close to each other with no blood ties but strong affective ones, families with single parents, ménages à trois or à quatre or more, and variations in family-like groupings that humans evolve in their quest for the best possible functional system for their needs. The student may have to cope with families with AIDS, incest, physical or sexual abuse, or fatal diseases.
- "Therapy": Supervision can help the trainee define his or her own style of helping families. The trainee can realize that therapy does not imply keeping a family together at all costs, nor seeking the impossible goal of producing a family without problems. Rather, it means helping the family find a way, a style, or a reconceptualization that will fit their values and their capacities and help

each member grow (if necessary, away from the original family unit that initiated treatment) to fulfill his or her potential. Therapy can only help the family achieve harmony in between crises and problem-solving dilemmas. Paying attention to these aspects of learning, the supervisor can provide the student with the conceptual, perceptual, and executive skills he or she needs to be an effective therapist (Cleghorn and Levin 1973; Tomm and Wright 1980).

When the family supervisor functions well, he or she will offer clarity of goals and skills, criticize constructively, trust the student, tolerate his or her mistakes (as long as they are progressively rectified), and tolerate constructive challenge and creative departures from his or her suggestions. The teacher must prepare the supervisee to fly solo.

When the supervisor does not function well, he or she may offer a confusing stance about goals and skills, teach in an arrogant or intolerant way, fail to show trust in the student or acceptance of correctable mistakes, and fail to welcome the supervisee's creative ideas that depart from the supervisor's own teaching. Another dysfunctional way of supervising is to offer only abstract musings that do not provide the student with advice on what to do with a specific family situation.

Family therapy supervisors need support as well. To this end, at Mount Sinai Hospital, a group of supervisors meets on a regular basis to discuss issues related to the supervision of psychiatric residents in family therapy. The meeting is multidisciplinary and includes family therapists with backgrounds in psychiatry, nursing, and social work. This allows supervisors to solve territoriality conflicts, prevents a sense of isolation, and provides support for dealing with problems that arise in the course of supervision. It also permits supervisors to teach each other and share what they have learned from their students.

Because of many factors, family therapy is still relatively undervalued and undertaught as a modality, particularly in adult psychiatric settings. We at Mount Sinai Hospital believe a family systems perspective is an indispensable tool in the psychiatrist's armamentarium.

Through a family therapy seminar program and through supervision, we have endeavored to carve a niche in our residents' minds. We hope to make family therapy a modality with which trainees will feel comfortable and use naturally when they deem it appropriate in their psychiatric practices. We also hope that some of them will become interested enough in the field to undertake a full program of specialization in family therapy elsewhere.

References

Andolfi M, Menghi P: A model for training in family therapy, in Dimensions of Family Therapy. Edited by Andolfi M, Menghi P. New York, Guilford, 1980, pp 239–259

Berger M, Dammann C: Live supervision as context, treatment and training. Fam Process 21:337–344, 1982

Bertalanffy L von: General Systems Theory: Foundation, Development, Applications. New York, Braziller, 1968

Bodin A: Videotape applications to training family therapists. J Nerv Ment Dis 148:251–262, 1969

Burdill DR: The simulated family as an aid to learning family group treatment. Child Welfare 55:703–709, 1976

Chagoya L: Difficulties in teaching and learning family therapy [in Spanish]. Psiquiatría (Mexico) 5:23–29, 1975

Chagoya L: Family psychotherapy [in Spanish], in Manual de Psiquiatría. Edited by Rivera JLG, Vela A, Arana J. Madrid, Spain, Editorial Karpos, 1980, pp 1048–1054

Chagoya L: An eclectic approach to family therapy [black & white videotape]. Hamilton, Ontario, McMaster University, 1983

Cleghorn JM, Levin S: Training family therapists by setting learning objectives. Am J Orthopsychiatry 43:439–446, 1973

Cornwell M, Pearson R: Cotherapy teams and one-way screen in family therapy training. Fam Process 20:199–209, 1981

De Shazer S, Berg IK, Lipchnik E, et al: Brief therapy: focused solution development. Fam Process 25:207–221, 1986

Erikson EH: Identity, Youth and Crisis. New York, WW Norton, 1968

Gershenson J, Cohen MS: Through the looking glass: the experiences of two family therapy trainees with live supervision. Fam Process 17:225–230, 1978

Liddle HA, Breunlin DC, Schwartz RC (eds): Handbook of Family Therapy Training and Supervision. New York, Guilford, 1988

Mansfield F: Supervised role-play in the teaching of the process of consultation. Med Educ 25:485–490, 1991

McDaniel SH, Weber I, McKeever J: Multiple theoretical approaches to supervision: choices in family therapy training. Fam Process 22:491–500, 1983

McGoldrick M, Carter EA: The family life-cycle, in Normal Family Processes. Edited by Walsh F. New York, Guilford, 1982, pp 167–195

Nichols MP: The Self in the System: Expanding the Limits of Family Therapy. New York, Brunner/Mazel, 1987

Scharff DE, Savege Scharff J: Object Relations Family Therapy. Northvale, NJ, Jason Aronson, 1987

Schwartz RC: The trainer-trainee relationship in family therapy training, in Handbook of Family Therapy Training and Supervision. Edited by Liddle HA, Breunlin DC, Schwartz RC. New York, Guilford, 1988, pp 172–182

Steinhauer PD, Santa-Barbara J, Skinner J: The process model of family functioning. Can J Psychiatry 29:77–88, 1984

Tomm KM, Wright LM: Training in family therapy: perceptual, conceptual and executive skills. Fam Process 18:227–250, 1980

Watzlawick P, Beavin JH, Jackson DD: Pragmatics of Human Communication. New York, WW Norton, 1967

Wheeler D, Myers Avis J, Miller LA, et al: Rethinking family therapy training and supervision: a feminist model, in Women in Families: A Framework for Family Therapy. Edited by McGoldrick C, Anderson M, Walsh F. New York, WW Norton, 1989, pp 139–151

Whiffen R, Byng-Hall J (eds): Family Therapy Supervision: Recent Developments in Practice. New York, Grune & Stratton, 1982

Whitaker CA, Keith DV: Symbolic-experiential family therapy, in Handbook of Family Therapy. Edited by Gurman AS, Kniskern DP. New York, Brunner/Mazel, 1981, pp 221–224

White M: Negative explanation, restrained and double description: a template for family therapy. Fam Process 25:169–184, 1986

Chapter 9

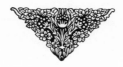

Supervision of Patients With Recurrent Psychosis

Mary V. Seeman, M.D., F.R.C.P.C., and
Melvin Prosen, M.D., F.R.C.P.C.*

T his chapter is intended for both supervisees and supervisors. We discuss several critical issues invariably encountered when psychiatry residents work with that heterogeneous group of patients generally subsumed under the diagnosis of schizophrenia. The data base from which our emphasis emerges is the now-faded recollection of psychiatric residency some 30 years ago and our subsequent long and varied experience in the intensive treatment and supervision of patients in varying stages of psychosis. Many former patients are in sporadic contact with us, and their reconstructions of their treatment from years ago continue to startle, amaze, and instruct us.

When as residents we treated them in the hospital and in the clinic, they were, it seems, aware that their therapists were being "overseen" by some other "invisible, omniscient, omnipotent force" (i.e., the supervisor). It is difficult, in retrospect, to calculate the ramifications

---

*Dr. Prosen died on October 2, 1992, shortly after completing his work on this chapter.

of that intuitive knowledge and how much (influenced as it must have been by our own personal struggles with our supervisors) it affected these patients, for good or for ill. Whatever else these old struggles achieved, they aroused our interest in the supervisor-therapist-patient triad, especially as applied to the treatment of individuals with schizophrenia.

Over the intervening years, both of us have supervised many psychiatry residents ourselves and have become increasingly aware of the problems of the supervisor, especially of his or her divided loyalties as facilitator, evaluator, administrator, and arm's-length clinician. Although these same multiple roles are assumed by all supervisors, situations that arise in the treatment of severely ill, psychotic individuals test these separate loyalties with particular intensity.

Over the years, we have also had occasion to speak with scores of residents about their supervision experiences. What we have learned is that a resident's perspective on psychotherapy and on humanity is very much shaped by the attitudes of his or her supervisors, not so much by what they say but by what they do or refrain from doing. One *apparent* conclusion is that very few supervisors value the humanity of the person whose affliction happens to be schizophrenia. Very few psychiatry residents are encouraged to spend "quality time" with their schizophrenia patients. Psychotherapy supervisors, almost without exception, prefer to supervise residents on treatment sessions with patients whose problems are considered less severe.

It is our hope that the discussion in this chapter will facilitate the psychotherapeutic treatment of the patient with recurrent psychosis. The psychotic patient lives in a world that is "sublime" (i.e., inexpressible, fantastic, frightening, ecstatic, awesome [Bowers and Freedman 1966; Buckley 1981]), and the beginning therapist inevitably gets embroiled in this world, dragging the sometimes reluctant and perhaps overly conservative supervisor behind. Heroic odysseys—marked with temptations, dangers, impossible challenges, somber outlooks, and the ultimate small victories—await this patient-therapist-supervisor triad along the difficult course of treatment and supervision.

Person Versus Case

Medical teaching has a way of dehumanizing patients and turning them into cases: cases of diabetes, cases of kidney failure, cases of schizophrenia. Much has been written about this process and about how, as reprehensible as it is, it serves understandable defensive purposes. It helps the medical student deal with what could otherwise overwhelm him or her: the powerful emotions elicited by illness, dependency, helplessness, and death. Psychiatry training needs to undo some of what medical school has done, but it does not always succeed.

In the United States and Canada, many psychiatric residency programs do not provide sufficient informed faculty to teach the fundamental skills of supportive psychotherapy, so necessary in the complex therapeutic relatedness that is established with regressed patients (Everett 1989; Frances 1989; Magder 1984). Although psychiatry trainees are taught to be vigilant to the effect they are having on their patients and to the patients' impact on them, patients with schizophrenia are exempted from this guiding principle. Such a patient is treated briefly or in large groups, delegated to the care of "case managers," and *managed* rather than treated. As a result, the treatment philosophy of a caring, sensitive, humane interaction seems to have been abandoned in the interventions offered to these patients. Psychotherapy (and psychotherapy supervision) are reserved for more psychologically minded patients. This, then, becomes the first issue in beginning supervision with a schizophrenia patient: what is it about the person with schizophrenia, *this* person with schizophrenia, that makes the trainee elect to see the "schizophrenia" and overlook the person?

> *Resident:* I wouldn't do therapy with a schizophrenic patient because schizophrenic symptoms don't respond to therapy.

> *Supervisor:* Would you do therapy with a person who has a cold? . . . Yet the symptoms of a cold won't respond to therapy either.

This redefinition of the intent and direction of psychotherapy—toward the person rather than toward symptoms—is important and can be effectively taught by directing students to study the subjective experience of their patients. A useful tool for the supervisor is the reading list. This list should include accounts of patients' own experiences such as those of A Recovering Patient (1986) and Anonymous (1989). Volume 15 of the *Schizophrenia Bulletin,* in which the latter article appears, is devoted entirely to the topic of subjective experiences in schizophrenia.

> *Resident:* I wouldn't do therapy with a schizophrenic patient because getting close will make the patient worse.

> *Supervisor:* Getting close could make any person feel worse if it's done against his or her wishes. A forced intimacy is usually unwelcome.

The issue of the *frame* in the therapy of a patient with schizophrenia is an important one for both supervisor and resident to explore at the beginning of their relationship and at the beginning of the resident's relationship with the patient. Frame refers to issues of therapeutic distance, scheduling, pace of therapy, therapeutic attitude, privacy, confidentiality, time-keeping, extra appointments, missed sessions, office arrangements, therapists' absences, and consistency of response to home phone calls or to questions of a personal nature asked of the therapist. These issues, which are significant in all therapeutic encounters, need to be rethought in the context of the vulnerable patient and perhaps made more flexible than they might otherwise be. Residents may, however, confuse flexibility with inconsistency. The important difference between these attitudes and subsequent behaviors needs repeated consideration and role-modeling by the supervisor.

The optimal therapeutic distance for patients with schizophrenia is defined as consistent friendliness, kindliness, understanding, and acceptance, without unprofessional closeness (McGlashan 1983). A similar distance needs to be adopted between resident and supervisor. It is very difficult to maintain one sort of distance with the supervisor, whether more distant or more close, and another with the patient who is being discussed. Compiling the literature on intensive individual psychotherapy with schizophrenia patients, McGlashan (1983) further counsels a distance "close enough to give but not to scare" (p. 917). He cites others in suggesting that the most serious drawback to effectiveness is the therapist's need to be liked. The same could be said of the supervisor. To maintain an appropriate distance with a trainee, a supervisor must forego the temptation of wanting to be "friends."

McGlashan (1983) also emphasizes the need to be reliable with the psychotic patient (i.e., to start and stop appointments on time). By extension, this is also essential for the supervisor. Pace is an attribute related to distance. Pace with the psychotic patient needs to be slow enough to leave time to measure the helpfulness (or not) of a specific intervention. Supervision of the resident also proceeds best when the pace is leisurely, contemplative, and unhurried.

Attention to issues of therapeutic frame, as these need to be adjusted to the requirements of special patients, will remove the attribution of "nonpersonhood" from these patients and will serve the resident well throughout his or her training and future career.

Control Versus Understanding

Listening to violent and erotic fantasies in nonpsychotic patients does not, as a rule, arouse undue anxiety in therapist or supervisor. At leisure, they figure out together the *why now* and the *why this* of the patient's preoccupation. The situation is markedly different when the patient has been psychotic, when he or she has demonstrated in the past that fantasy world and everyday world overlap. Under these circumstances, the therapist is usually made profoundly uncomfortable, worries for the patient, worries for the patient's possible victims, and worries about the extent of his or her own responsibility. The therapist is also concerned about his or her relationships with the patient, the patient's family, and the supervisor. He or she will struggle with ambivalent feelings ("should I intervene or should I not?") and with uncertainty. When are fantasies to be taken as precursors to behavior? When does behavior need to be controlled? Are the functions of understanding and limit setting somehow antithetical to each other?

> *Resident:* The patient was very upset. He said that whenever he spoke to his daughter on the phone, he could hear "them" mak-

ing noises in the walls. He figures "they" don't want him talking to his daughter. I think he's very delusional. I think I need to increase his medication. I told him that it must be hard talking to his daughter, missing her and wanting to see her, and her being so far away. He said, no, it would be fine talking to her if "they" left him alone. He thinks "they" want to give him the message not to talk to her. I said maybe he needs more medication to drown out the messages.

Supervisor: Your guess is that "they" are hostile, from the patient's viewpoint?

Resident: I don't know.

Supervisor: If "they" are friendly, in other words, if the messages are meant as guidance, does he want them drowned out?

Resident: But they're a symptom of illness, so it's my responsibility to make them go away, right? Even if they're friendly.

This is the second important issue in the treatment and supervision of psychotic patients: Does a "symptom" in the patient that gets transformed into a corresponding "symptom" in the clinician (e.g., fear of irrationality and the need to control it) inevitably lead to a "symptom" in the supervisor (e.g., intolerance of trial and error on the part of the resident and the need to control *it*)? In other words, should the supervisor tell the resident not to use medication too hastily, or should he or she perceive the resident's motive as "friendly" to the patient and not interfere unduly by insisting on what the supervisor thinks is clinically correct? Will the resident learn more from being told not to interfere with the patient, or would he or she learn more from the noninterfering stance of the supervisor?

Psychotic patients stimulate intense countertransference reactions. This is inevitable and ubiquitous. The patient may resonate with some regressive, primitive quality that resides in the most "healthy" of therapists. The supervisor must pay attention to these signposts and use this valuable information to help the therapist tolerate the patient's intense affects.

High doses and unusual combinations of medications are often clues to negative countertransference. This can be approached by the supervisor on the level of theoretical discussion about the pros and cons of medication adjustment in schizophrenia patients (Seeman 1990). Reading material about the efficacy of nonpharmacological interventions is appreciated by most trainees (Rappaport et al. 1978; Rosberg and Stunden 1990).

Patients' delusions are, of course, not always harmless. The situation with the patient could proceed in this direction.

> *Resident:* The patient came in with a black eye. Apparently he decided that his neighbor to the left was responsible for the wall noises, and he went next door and yelled at him and got punched out. The guy next door happens to be German and the patient has a thing about Germans, so it makes sense why he's focusing on him. The black eye is proof, he says, that the German neighbor is evil. Now he's planning his revenge. I get the impression that you think I overreact to these threats, so I just let him talk about it without interfering.
>
> *Supervisor:* Talking about it is not enough. You and I have to decide what to do about this, and you and the patient have to agree on a safe course of action.

There are times when immediate directive action has to be taken. "Understanding" is not the same as laissez-faire. This distinction is particularly key in the treatment and supervision of psychotic patients. McGlashan (1983) recommends tolerance of the bizarre and the confusing, but absolute firmness when it comes to potential violence. This firmness needs to be unequivocally communicated by the supervisor in word, tone of voice, and action.

Subjective Meaning

The therapy of psychotic patients often involves the substitution of the therapist's more benign meaning of events for the patient's meaning, which may be terrifying. To do this well, the clinician has to first realize that a wide gulf separates his or her understanding from the patient's understanding.

Resident: The patient is noncompliant.

Supervisor: To what?

Resident: To treatment.

Supervisor: Which treatment?

Resident: He won't take his meds. He says they interfere with his sex life. I think he's just denying his illness. He doesn't have a sex life. He admits he doesn't even *want* a sex life. Then he says he won't take his meds because of imagined sexual problems he doesn't even give himself a chance to have.

Supervisor: Let's look at those three concepts: meds, sex life, illness. I bet you and I may not always agree on what we mean by them. Do you think the patient and you are referring to the same thing?

Whereas different interpretations of the same word may occur with respect to any word or concept, misunderstandings with the patient are especially likely when it comes to medical jargon. The supervisor and resident may fall into the trap of validating each other's concept of what a word means (e.g., "schizophrenia") and forget that, for the patient, the word means something quite different (Fabrega 1987; Jones et al. 1983; Rabkin 1972; Rhodes 1984). In the same way, patient and resident, or patient and supervisor, may share private meanings based on common background, shared experience, or similar age, leaving the third party out in the cold. The significance of investigating shared meanings is especially important in working with psychotic patients who, by definition, live in a reality of their own.

Family Concerns

The young patient with schizophrenia brings his or her parents into treatment—not only in the introjected sense—but in the literal sense. Mother and/or father are always calling the therapist—to voice concerns, to ask questions, to give advice, to complain, to admonish. The patient may or may not approve of or even know about the calls. What should the therapist do? With nonpsychotic patients, he or she invokes principles of autonomy and confidentiality. With psychotic patients, the issues are different. Are the calls interference or collaboration? Are families part of the problem or part of the solution?

> *Resident:* They never leave well enough alone. They always expect more from him. They should be glad he's coming to his sessions. Now they want to know if he has discussed his school situation. They want me to know he's not sleeping. They're worried he's getting depressed. They're driving me crazy.

> *Supervisor:* For a while there, I didn't know you were talking about the family; I thought you were talking about you and me. That's exactly what *we* were concerned with last week—that he was depressed and not keeping up at school.

The triad of patient, therapist, and supervisor sometimes becomes so enmeshed that outside influences (i.e., families in this case) are resented. With psychotic patients, it is important to resist the inclination to therapeutic insularity. Others, especially families, are a potential source of extra help for the patient (Mintz et al. 1987; Seeman 1988; Thornton et al. 1982), and both resident and supervisor can help each other resist the temptation to shut the family out. Families, especially mothers, have often been unjustly blamed in the illness of their offspring. Psychoanalytic theories have been misapplied, and families have incurred the blame and shame of a child's unusual development. In these instances, the younger psychiatrist (the resident) may often take the lead in helping the older psychiatrist (the supervisor) question and change long-held attitudes about the role of the family in schizophrenia. This reversal of roles is one of the joys of supervision. It is a way for older psychiatrists to keep abreast of progress in the field and to give younger psychiatrists an opportunity to teach their elders. It also sets an example for the therapist who might consequently feel it is permissible to learn from patients.

Cotherapy

What was said in the preceding section about families also applies to cotherapists (i.e., social workers, psychologists, nurses, vocational counselors, occupational therapists, and others involved in the care of the schizophrenia patient). The resident therapist may fail to appreciate the roles other therapists play in the treatment of his patient. The supervisor's temptation might be to support the resident and collude with him or her in devaluing the work of others. The challenge for the supervisor is to support the resident while simultaneously acknowledging and appreciating the collective team approach (Seeman et al. 1982).

Mirroring Transference and Countertransference

When the patient is a nonconformist, as the psychotic patient always is, the supervisor can expect a rebellious supervisee who will want to try new things and do them in new ways. As we have mentioned, whenever the therapist is inclined to impose order on the patient's flights of fancy, the supervisor may find him- or herself critically reprimanding the therapist. When the patient is apathetic and unconnected, as patients with schizophrenia may often be, the therapist may appear distant and unmotivated to the supervisor and may elicit a volley of concrete suggestions on technique. This, of course, parallels the therapist's exasperation with the patient and attempts to "fill the patient's empty life" with concrete suggestions on what to do with his or her time.

These kinds of mirrorings occur throughout supervision. For instance, the patient basks in the high regard of the therapist; the therapist delights in the patient. The therapist, sure that all is going well, is open and enthusiastic with the supervisor. The supervisor is proud of the trainee and gives him or her a good evaluation. The therapist's confidence grows. This is communicated to the patient, who feels secure and in good hands. The patient then opens up and deals effectively with his or her ghosts. As can be seen, this is a circular process. It can start anywhere and produce good results all around. Sometimes it goes the other way, and everything progressively deteriorates. This is a constant danger when the patient is a severely ill, interpersonally awkward person, ever wary of therapeutic contact.

When one of us (M.V.S.) was a resident 30 years ago and one of the patients left treatment or otherwise "misbehaved," the supervisor insisted that the patient was merely acting out the unconscious rebellion of therapist against supervisor. Although this may have been accurate, these "accusations" are hurtful, rather than helpful. Inasmuch as the interpretation of mirroring can reduce anxiety, it is a potent explanatory principle. Used wrongly, it can steer beginning therapists away from doing therapy—or, at least, away from certain supervisors.

Hospitalization

The need for rehospitalization is always a possibility with psychotic patients. It does not constitute a failure of treatment. Some therapists hold such unrealistic expectations of themselves and their patients that they even construe a visit to the emergency room during the course of treatment as a failure of therapy. They may fear that their supervisors will criticize them for having permitted an exacerbation of illness. In addition, emergency care or hospital admission may increase unwelcome family involvement. It may require supplementary multidisciplinary team meetings, or that a new hospital team will take over the patient's care and exclude the treating resident. The resident may feel unsure of what his or her role now becomes, whether or not he or she continues to see the patient.

The supervisor's role in these circumstances is clear. He or she must focus the resident's attention on the crisis in the patient's life. The sequelae of hospitalization may preoccupy the resident, who must be guided back to the patient. What were the circumstances that triggered this relapse? Understanding the crisis will make its associated difficulties worthwhile.

Sometimes it falls to the therapist to have to admit the patient involuntarily to hospital. This is perhaps the ultimate understanding versus control situation (Applebaum and Hamm 1982). Most therapists in training find the involuntary certification of a patient they have been treating a very difficult task. The supervisor's support and guidance are much needed during this time of stress. Psychotic transference may need to be diluted through hospitalization. This represents a true psychiatric emergency, and the decision to certify may need to be taken without the supervisor's prior agreement. The supervisor may, of course, feel that the resident's decision was therapeutically wrong. As stated by McGlashan (1983), decisions such as these must be based on the therapist's level of anxiety and cannot be second-guessed by another person. The resident's anxiety can be explored as a separate issue.

Suicide

The ultimate in stress—and not so uncommon when dealing with schizophrenia patients—is attempted or completed suicide by the patient. The therapist is then faced with feelings about the loss of the patient, the anguish and blame directed at him or her by the family and perhaps the treatment team, the critical appraisal of the supervisor, the anger at the patient or others he or she feels are responsible, and—most of all—the conscience-stricken ruminations of what could have or should have been done (Brown 1987a, 1987b; Brownstein 1992; Caldwell and Gottesman 1990; Chemtob et al. 1988; Goldstein and Buongiorno 1984; Jacobs and Brown 1989; Kaye and Soreff 1991; Kolodny et al. 1979; Litman 1965). The supervisor must be there not only to listen and support but also to share some of the tasks that are an invariable accompaniment of suicide: continuing meetings with the family, conferences with the treating team, meetings with police and lawyers, and attendance at the inquest. Being there with the resident is perhaps the single best act of solidarity the supervisor can provide. Discussing personal experiences in dealing with patient suicides can be helpful to trainees. They need to know that roughly one-third of residents have a patient who commits suicide during the training years (Kaye and Soreff 1991). More than 50% of practicing psychiatrists have had that experience (Chemtob et al. 1988).

The suicide of patients early on in training can become a deterrent to subsequent close involvement. It hurts too much to try again, and the young resident may find him- or herself avoiding certain kinds of patients or certain kinds of being with patients. The supervisor, having probably been through this, is in the right position to inter-vene and convert this emotionally draining experience into one the resident will want to risk again.

Separation and Termination

Patient suicides occur, as often as not, at the time of resident change-over. The 6-month or 1-year turnover of psychiatric residents plays havoc with patients' feelings and may set off a series of reactions that end tragically. Seasoned supervisors are attuned to this but not always able to prevent it. Residents working with chronically ill pa-tients often undervalue their significance to these individuals. It is important that they skillfully terminate and remain especially vigilant to apparent apathy and silence masking a distorted grief reaction. This needs to be well attended to or it will undermine beneficial work with the next therapist. One frequently repeated error is for the resident to reduce the dose of antipsychotic medication just be-fore terminating with the patient. The reduced medication dose is a symbol of the patient's having improved and is a parting gift the patient and resident exchange. Unfortunately, the timing is wrong. The meaning of medication dose changes is a fruitful topic of resi-dent/supervisor discussion. An actual exchange of gifts is much to be preferred over symbolic gestures that may be harmful. The super-visor may lead the way by giving the resident a going-away gift that is concrete rather than symbolic.

Residents also have their own separation difficulties: separation from the patient and separation from the supervisor. The mentor relationship becomes particularly strong when the patient is severely disturbed. This is because the trainee and the supervisor are forced to work together and to solve many upsetting and difficult problems. Preventive work preparatory to the separation anxiety that accompanies termination can be done before supervisor or super-visee vacations. Vacations are excellent training exercises. Learning to exchange postcards during these times sets the stage for being able to keep in touch afterward, when the therapeutic relationship and the supervisory relationship are over.

Summary

Special issues arise in the supervision of therapy with psychotic patients. Several of these have been covered in this chapter. The first task of the supervisor is to delineate for the trainee the distinction between the person with schizophrenia and the effects of schizophrenia on the person. Pace, structure, and optimal distance within the supervisory relationship serve as models for the trainee in evolving his or her relationship with the patient. A nondirective stance on the part of the supervisor will facilitate tolerance on the part of the therapist for the patient's confused thinking and sometimes bizarre behavior. Violence, on the other hand, must never be tolerated, and it is the supervisor's responsibility to intervene immediately when the line between fantasy and threat of violence is breached.

Shared meanings are especially significant in the treatment and supervision of psychotic patients. They bind individuals together but may also serve to shut a person out if the meanings are too idiosyncratic. Family concerns, multidisciplinary team issues, and the limits of confidentiality are recurring supervisory topics. Transference/countertransference reactions and their parallels in the supervision relationship are important learning opportunities. Hospitalization, suicide threats, and the meaning of neuroleptic dose changes have been given special consideration here. Separation issues have been emphasized, as they are particularly meaningful in the treatment of schizophrenia patients. Most important of all is the supervisor's role in allowing the therapist to experience the excitement and potential of working with psychotic patients without being frightened away by the difficulties of the task.

References

Anonymous: First person account: a delicate balance. Schizophr Bull 15:345–346, 1989

Applebaum PS, Hamm RM: Decision to seek commitment. Arch Gen Psychiatry 39:447–451, 1982

A Recovering Patient: "Can we talk?": the schizophrenic patient in psychotherapy. Am J Psychiatry 143:68–70, 1986

Bowers MB Jr, Freedman DX: "Psychedelic" experiences in acute psychosis. Arch Gen Psychiatry 15:240–248, 1966

Brown HN: Patient suicide during residency training, I: incidence, implications, and program response. Journal of Psychiatric Education 11:201–216, 1987a

Brown HN: The impact of suicide on therapists in training. Compr Psychiatry 28:101–112, 1987b

Brownstein M: Contacting the family after a suicide. Can J Psychiatry 37:208–212, 1992

Buckley P: Mystical experience and schizophrenia. Schizophr Bull 7:516–521, 1981

Caldwell CB, Gottesman II: Schizophrenics kill themselves too: a review of risk factors for suicide. Schizophr Bull 16:571–589, 1990

Chemtob CM, Hamada RS, Bauer G, et al: Patients' suicides: frequency and impact on psychiatrists. Am J Psychiatry 145:224–228, 1988

Everett A: Labelling and persons with mental illness. Schizophr Bull 15:511–513, 1989

Fabrega H: Psychiatric diagnosis: a cultural perspective. J Nerv Ment Dis 175:383–394, 1987

Frances AJ: Foreword, in Schizophrenia: Treatment, Process and Outcome. Edited by McGlashan TH, Keats CJ. Washington, DC, American Psychiatric Press, 1989, pp xi–xiii

Goldstein LS, Buongiorno PA: Psychotherapists as suicide survivors. Am J Psychother 38:392–398, 1984

Jacobs D, Brown HN (eds): Suicide: Understanding and Responding. Madison, CT, International Universities Press, 1989

Jones W, Kahn M, MacDonald J: Psychiatric patients' views of mental illness, hospitalization, and treatment. J Nerv Ment Dis 136:82–87, 1983

Kaye NS, Soreff SM: The psychiatrist's role, responses, and responsibilities when a patient commits suicide. Am J Psychiatry 148:739–743, 1991

Kolodny S, Binder RL, Bronstein AA, et al: The working through of patients' suicides by four therapists. Suicide Life Threat Behav 9:33–46, 1979

Litman RE: When patients commit suicide. Am J Psychother 19:570–576, 1965

Magder D: Seeing the person behind the psychosis. Can Fam Physician Med Fam Can 30:369–372, 1984

McGlashan TH: Intensive individual psychotherapy of schizophrenia: a review of techniques. Arch Gen Psychiatry 40:909–920, 1983

Mintz LI, Liberman RP, Miklowitz DI, et al: Expressed emotion: a call for partnership among relatives, patients, and professionals. Schizophr Bull 227:235, 1987

Rabkin J: Opinions about mental illness: a review of the literature. Psychol Bull 77:153–171, 1972

Rappaport M, Hopkins HD, Hall K: Are these schizophrenics for whom drugs may be unnecessary or contraindicated? International Pharmacopsychiatry 13:100–111, 1978

Rhodes LA: "This will clear your mind": the use of metaphors for medication in psychiatric settings. Cult Med Psychiatry 8:49–70, 1984

Rosberg J, Stunden AA: The use of direct confrontation: the treatment resistant schizophrenic patient. Acta Psychiatr Scand 81:352–358, 1990

Seeman MV: The family and schizophrenia. Humane Medicine 4:96–101, 1988

Seeman MV: Antipsychotic medication, in Office Treatment of Schizophrenia. Edited by Seeman MV, Greben SE. Washington, DC, American Psychiatric Press, 1990, pp 123–139

Seeman MV, Pyke J, Denberg D, et al: Co-therapy in a schizophrenia clinic. Can J Psychiatry 27:296–300, 1982

Thornton JF, Plummer E, Seeman MV, et al: The family's reaction to schizophrenic illness. International Journal of Family Psychiatry 3:33–44, 1982

Chapter 10

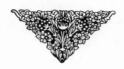

Emergency and Crisis Psychotherapy Supervision

Rodney Slonim, M.D., F.R.C.P.C.

In this chapter, I demonstrate how supervision of psychiatric residents in the emergency/crisis situation, based on a psychodynamic perspective, can help their therapeutic interventions become more effective. Through supervision, this demanding and somewhat anxiety-provoking area will no longer be seen as so burdensome. Rather, it can been seen as an opportunity to help in an active way, thereby dealing with the potential disillusionment that occurs so frequently in this area. The significant place of the psychotherapeutic perspective in understanding the crisis and its use in effecting the resolution of the emergency/crisis situation are also highlighted.

The growing shortage of inpatient beds both in Canadian and U.S. hospitals has increased the pressure on psychiatric residents to deal effectively with emergencies and crises. I view psychiatric emergencies and crises as states in which the individual's psychological capacity to deal with an internal and external event has been overwhelmed. My focus with the resident is to develop an understanding of the crisis as part of a continuum arising out of the characteristic personality style of that person, and to understand that vulnerability to crisis is essentially determined by how competent each person is at resolving previous neurotic conflicts and as well by the degree of ego intactness. Harris and colleagues (1963) have emphasized that a crisis is a dynamic structure in which a precipitating stress calls on the individual's repertoire of personality traits, characterological defenses, adaptive capacities, and unconscious conflicts. I believe that the essential element required in the supervisory relationship is the development of a perspective that reinforces the active psychotherapeutic stance in the emergency/crisis situation.

At first glance, this may appear to diminish the place of a psychodynamic psychoanalytic perspective. In reality, the *way* in which the therapist is active, both in his or her intellectual perspective and therapeutic stance—drawing on the reservoir of psychological understanding, empathic, intuitive responsiveness, and ultimately integrating all of this in the response to the person's crisis—reinforces the significant place of the psychodynamic perspective.

In addressing the supervisory relationship, I have found Glick and Meyerson's article (1980–1981) "The Use of Psychoanalytic Concepts in Crisis Intervention" to be particularly useful. The authors draw heavily upon Bibring's (1954) description of the technical procedures of suggestion, abreaction, manipulation, clarification, and interpretation.

Emergency/crisis intervention provides a unique teaching and learning opportunity in dealing with vital countertransference issues. The patient in crisis characteristically presents feeling overwhelmed, often confused, and needy—manifestations of the regressive experience with heightening of transference wishes. There is a sense of urgency and helplessness that affects the therapist intervention. This clinical presentation frequently can evoke a major countertransference response in the therapist—the unconscious identification with the helpless, childlike patient, which can lead to a variety of defensive responses, often involving fantasies of or wishes for omnipotent control—ultimately presenting in some cases as a grandiose rescue fantasy (Glick and Meyerson 1980–1981).

Another common countertransference response is passivity, a defensive manifestation that is potentially lethal in the face of a seriously suicidal patient.

In dealing with borderline or characterologically disturbed patients in the emergency/crisis situation, hostile and unempathic responses are particular countertransference reactions that often represent the therapist's defensive response to the powerful punitive and persecutory superego projections of the patient. In this intense context, the therapist's own unresolved conflicts may also be reactivated, particularly by patients who present with similar conflicts.

I present a series of clinical vignettes to illustrate the supervisory process and demonstrate some of these countertransference issues.

> A 55-year-old man who was a successful business executive presents to the emergency department feeling overwhelmed, anxious, depressed, and suicidal. He was facing a bowel resection and permanent colostomy for his recently diagnosed rectal carcinoma. Given that he recently established a meaningful relationship with a younger woman, and their sexual relationship was extremely important and satisfying for both of them, the realization that he faces a high risk of impotence following the surgery precipitated this acute suicidal presentation. He is now fearful that he will be abandoned and pitied by this woman. Having had a long history of failed relationships, including several marriages and a traumatic early childhood, he is feeling hopeless, and asks "What is the point in trying? I will only be alone once more."

The first-year resident in the supervisory session presented all the pertinent findings on this man: his helplessness, his depression and suicidal ideation, his fear of the loss of potency, his fear of the loss of his young girlfriend.

In this instance, a particularly insightful and introspective young male resident was able to present the above case and acknowledge his own feelings of anxiety, passivity, and helplessness in the face of the patient's overwhelming and understandable life concerns. The supervisor was able to listen empathically to and resonate with the resident's feelings that were stirred up by this patient, and to also become aware of the resident's immediate impulse to take control of this patient's life. Here the unconscious identification with the helpless, childlike presentation of the patient clearly led to a wish for omnipotent control as a defensive response to the resident's own feelings of helplessness and passivity. By exploring this with the resident, he was able to see that this represented for the patient a characteristic way of dealing with overwhelming crisis. Further history has demonstrated this behavior to be a lifelong pattern of the patient's based on feelings of shame and humiliation in the face of being abandoned at moments of trauma.

The resident, supported by the empathic listening and clarification in the supervisory process, finds this further enhances his own empathic listening to the patient's pain, fear, and dread—the parallel process. The resident was then able to point out to the patient that the patient's own concerns (i.e., his fear, passivity, and suicidal preoccupation) were understood as his inability to speak directly and openly with his partner about his illness. It was then suggested to this patient that he was not as helpless nor as much a victim as he believed. He was encouraged to speak to his significant other about his fears, in spite of his concern that she would leave him or pity him.

What was suggested to the patient was that his view of himself as a passive victim was inherently maladaptive and unobjective. His present feelings—precipitated by the sudden diagnosis of cancer—were linked to internal conflicts that, although unknown to him, were affecting his view of himself and his life. The therapist indicated to the patient that his anxiety would become more tolerable, and his helplessness would diminish as his underlying conflicts became clear.

Within the supervisory relationship, I have found the technical procedures that use Bibring's (1954) concepts of suggestion, abreaction, manipulation, clarification, and interpretation to be particularly helpful. Using such procedures, the resident was able to frame the process of manipulation—that is, he was able to help and encourage the patient to act in a way different from the patient's own expected behavior. Instead of assuming omnipotent control as a countertransference reaction, the resident was able to clearly communicate to the patient that "no decision need be made until you can make sense of and understand the nature of your crisis." This technical intervention was facilitating through both removing the obstacles to understanding and improving the patient's adjustment.

By utilizing clarification, the resident in the emergency/crisis situation is able to demonstrate by a coherent presentation to the patient the distortions that are contained in the patient's thoughts, feelings, and behavior. Within the supervisory relationship, understanding on the part of the supervisor (and sensitivity to the overwhelming aspects of these real life events for the patient, which stimulate similar feelings in the resident) provides a supportive and holding function for the resident and can thereby be used in a complementary fashion within the therapeutic relationship. Therefore, instead of a grandiose rescue fantasy that was first experienced by the resident, he then was able to organize and reflect back to the patient in a way that allowed for emergence of the patient's own self-observing capacities, with utilization of the auxiliary ego function and identification processes.

In our treatment setting, my colleagues and I have found Viederman's (1983) psychodynamic life narrative to be extremely useful in dealing with emergency/crisis states. Essentially, this is a statement made to the patient that gives meaning to his or her current emotional reaction, in the context of his or her life history, and shows it to be a logical and inevitable product of previous life experience. As Viederman states, it addresses three fundamental characteristics of the emergency/crisis state: psychic disequilibrium with chaos and confusion; regression with intensification of strong transference wishes; and the inclination to examine the trajectory of one's life as it relates to self-perception, past accomplishments, and future hopes and aspirations.

Although the latter characteristic is much more common in people with physical disability and/or depression, this has been modified in our setting to deal with a whole variety of clinical presentations. In the case of the patient just discussed, with careful review of his presentation and the empathic and clarifying responses within the supervisory relationship, the resident was able to construct a psychodynamic life narrative for the patient in the following manner.

> It seems [the resident told the patient] that all your life you have felt that somehow you are not worthy of or good enough to have the love of your mother, nor could you please her or your father, in spite of your academic success. You have always wished for that special person who would somehow restore to you a sense

of security and of being worthwhile. You have overcome adversity; you have quit your compulsive gambling; you have restored your business with much success and are involved once more in a loving relationship. It seems that no matter what the adversity, you have been able to master it. Now with the prospect of surgery and permanent colostomy, you feel again like that humiliated and ashamed little boy of 5, who is forced by external circumstances to submit to a humiliating experience beyond your control.

The patient remembered being left in a sandbox at age 5 by his mother, who became preoccupied and did not respond to his entreaties of needing to use the bathroom. Finally, he was unable to control himself any longer. He wet himself and then was humiliated by his mother's screaming response to his "willful act." The resident went on to tell him:

The uncertainty of what this cancer brings is also a constant undercurrent that forces you to face your own mortality for the first time.

The reason for living is now firmly thrust in front of you and you are reevaluating your life, your purpose, and your present relationship. Clearly, your past behavior and actions have always represented a basic belief in yourself that has carried you through past adversities. Although you are afraid of being rejected and alone, you have not discussed this with your girlfriend. You are afraid that she will respond like your mother and your previous lovers and wives. Yet this concern can only be answered by a frank discussion with her.

You are not alone. You have told us that there are people who care for you, and we will be here to help you through this difficult time.

The patient settled in in response to this and returned for ongoing therapy following referral to a therapist in the outpatient department. Having discussed frankly with his significant other what he was facing, to his surprise she was supportive and did not abandon him. The resident, by virtue of recognizing his own countertransference reactions that had been stimulated by the patient's regressive transference manifestations, was able to use this experience. He understood the transference availability and readiness of the patient in an emergency/crisis situation to be a vital component that can make the therapist's activities therapeutically significant for the patient. In this sense, the transference availability and readiness of the resident to the supervisor, based on unconscious identification with the patient, was the process upon which the appropriate intervention was based.

Greenacre (1975) and Stone (1961) have elaborated on the fundamental or primary transference. They believe that this is a substrate upon which all effective psychotherapeutic interventions rest. Their concept implies that patients who are capable of entering usefully into therapy have developed in their life experiences (particularly in the mother/child dyad) a background of sufficient trust for the establishment of an object relationship during therapy, or in fact for any meaningful relationship, that will enable the therapy, the therapeutic encounter, and the relationship to develop.

As Viederman (1983) puts it: "A trusting and protective umbrella with this developmental origin is a prerequisite for intimate object relations and is a background for all meaningful psychotherapeutic relationships" (p. 243). With his patient, by presenting a narrative that spanned his life, the resident was able to convey to him a sense of having known him over time. As Viederman states, "Like the good parent who has a perspective on the child, what is captured in this life narrative is a quality of a shared experience over time" (p. 243). Thus the resident becomes, in the emergency/crisis situation, a reassuring parental figure. This conveys to the patient a sense of hope and protection. The resident is able to fully appreciate the essential aspect of support within the psychotherapeutic relationship. He or she therefore has had a unique opportunity in this emergency/crisis situation to provide this communicated understanding.

By clarifying for the resident the regression in this patient's coping capacity and ego adaptation to an earlier, more childlike mode in which the patient feels overwhelmed and helpless, the supervisor can demonstrate the sense of fluidity of the emergency/crisis situation. The patient has positive wishes for help from the resident,

which involve intensified dependency strivings along with the corre-
lated idealization of powerful parental figures. Supervisors have a
similar opportunity to use the complementary dynamic in developing
and clarifying the transference parameters within the supervisory
process as well. This demonstrates in an understandable and useful
way the transference readiness that is apparent in the majority of
emergency/crisis patients.

With a psychodynamic narrative, not only is a resident taken in
(so to speak), but the resident's construct is also taken in and assim-
ilated under the powerful influence of an idealizing transference that
increases the ego's integrative capacity. These are important concep-
tualizations that come alive in the process of supervision and are
useful in demonstrating to the resident an appreciation of the psychodynamic perspective in dealing with these patients. The parallel
process that ultimately complements the resident's own intervention
with the patient is a living, exciting, and gratifying experience.

> A 43-year-old divorced professional woman presented to the
> emergency room with anxiety, panic attacks, and a fear of dis-
> integrating. In the interview room, she turned to the examiners
> and said: "I can't stand being here. I don't like this room, and I
> don't like this bed here [pointing to a couch located near her
> chair]." Further history reveals verbal abuse and abandonment
> by an idealized alcoholic mother and sexual abuse by her step-
> father, which occurred from the ages of 5 to 16. The patient was
> fearful and mistrustful of the resident, who happened to be a
> senior resident in his last year of the program.

In this instance, the resident was able to contrast the situation in
which, instead of an idealizing transference in a patient with a basic
nurturing trust founded in the earlier unconscious memory of fundamental transference, he is confronted with a patient whose idealization is based on a more primitive idealization. Instead of seeing an
early gratifying relationship with an integrated good object, the resident sees a traumatic relationship with a fragmented, nonintegrated,
split good/bad object.

Here is an opportunity to work within the supervisory process and to develop with the resident a clear picture of these patients with character disorders who often present as help rejectors. In this case, help is ambivalently sought and then rejected with equal ambivalence. Such patients represent a discrete clinical group characterized by a common symptom profile, a similar treatment history, and a typical style interacting with the therapist-resident that is usually described as negativistic, demanding, and manipulative. There often is a paucity of social and interpersonal supports, and these patients tend to leave the emergency staff, like others, exhausted (Kahn 1984). In fact, this exhaustion and frustration with them often is conveyed to the resident by the emergency staff in somewhat hostile and distancing ways, such as "You get this patient out of here; this is your problem, and this patient is taking up too much of our time."

This is an important opportunity for the supervisor to share with the resident that this is a protracted process of engagement and containment—with frequent flights from the helper, which is in a sense the patient's psychodynamic life narrative. These patients have difficulty in tolerating limits. They experience distance as abandonment and closeness as entrapment, and the therapeutic space is fragile. They engender a great deal of discomfort in the therapist-resident, and countertransference feelings run high because of the powerful projective identifications. All these concepts are significant as theoretical considerations and dynamic organizations that become available within the supervisory space. They are useful in helping the resident understand and treat these difficult patients.

What is important for the supervisor to remember and to underline with the resident is that the patient's interaction is a reflection of his or her earlier developmental problems. A stance of empathy, rather than provocation, is important. A supportive and operant approach that reinforces the patient's appropriate behavior and cooperativeness and effects understanding, while improving or setting limits on demanding or inappropriate behavior, can be effective (Kahn 1984). In this case, the resident, although senior, had chosen a more biologically oriented career and, although he was familiar with psychodynamic principles, was not comfortable in dealing with a patient who was rejecting and somewhat hostile and frightened.

In his presentation to the supervisor, the resident experienced some frustration and anger and an unsettling amount of anxiety that he could not quite put his finger on. It was clear that the patient's perception of the couch in the emergency interview room as a bed raised concerns and anxieties in the resident as a potential sexual innuendo. He described her behavior as somewhat seductive and was quite concerned about her potential for disintegration.

Within the supervisory setting, the projective identification of the patient to the resident as a victimizing, sexually exploitive, and rejecting parent was empathically clarified, which relieved the resident's anxieties and made him comfortable enough to reveal what he felt was a rather harsh tone in responding to her. It was suggested that this perhaps was his method of creating some distance from his feeling threatened by her presentation and concerned about intensifying her fragility. The resident had an opportunity to explore the potential emergence of regressive wishes for sadistic attack that could follow the frustration of all of his intended therapeutic activity. Glick and Meyerson (1980–1981) have described such positions as manifested by intrusive questioning, verbal harassment, or retaliatory rejection that may lurk under the guise of judicious limit setting. These are characteristic of countertransference reactions. Because many of these patients are experienced as being frustrating to all who deal with them, and because they seem to be seeking the satisfaction of attack, rejection, and victimization, they are quite successful in provoking these countertransferential responses in a defensive way from therapists in general.

Upon clarifying the countertransference/transference dyad, and by virtue of the empathic understanding of the resident's own anxiety and fearfulness that are part of the response to the powerful projective identification by this patient, the resident was able to interpret her basic mistrust of him as her fear of men, never interpreting the unconscious wish for involvement. The patient settled in when, upon further exploration, her anxiety about being a good mother to her 13-year-old son was addressed. The fact that her son was described as seductive with her was simply noted, and she was referred for further treatment. Here, the significance of the symbol "bed-couch" and understanding the role of her early experience, basic mistrust, and anxiety were crucial.

This case offered the resident and the supervisor an opportunity to discuss and explore "symbolism," which provided insight into the crisis as well as potential therapeutic maneuvers.

Conversely, because the therapist-resident may overreact defensively to the grandiose rescue fantasy and become concerned about taking too much control out of the patient's hands, he or she may fall prey to *underactivity*.

Patients in emergency/crisis situations evoke a multiplicity of feelings, both realistic and transferential. Understanding these feelings is crucial, but the therapist-resident must not be overcome by self-preoccupation that results in action. Inexperienced therapists-residents (and that includes all of us to some degree) often waver between being totally drawn into acting for the patient or letting the patient flounder helplessly.

I agree with Talbott (1980–1981), who encourages errors on the side of overinvolvement. Talbott argues that a therapist may always analyze overenthusiasm but may not so easily be able to recover from the patient's loss of functioning.

> An 80-year-old married woman was brought to the emergency room by her daughters and husband, following an attempted overdose. Although she had had one episode of depression 40 years before when she discovered her husband's infidelity, she had been relatively well until the present time. Her house had recently been sold, and she and her husband were about to move into a condominium. She presented with extreme denial but agreed to admission at the urging of her daughters and the resident.
>
> A bed was not available and the resident decided not to press for it nor to call the backup supervisor to intervene. Upon hearing the presentation of the case even with the understanding that the patient was to be admitted the following morning, the supervisor urged her immediate admission and spoke to the chief of service to arrange this. Upon admission, and before the staff psychiatrist interviewed the patient, the patient hung herself from a shower but survived.

What alerted the supervisor to this urgent and potentially fatal outcome? In discussion with the resident about the complexities of this case, the supervisor became concerned about the patient's extreme denial. Even in the face of apparent family support, significant changes in the patient's life and her preoccupation with suicide raised this concern in the light of the long history of denial, rationalization, and apparently "normal" functioning, because of the disruption and significant losses that this woman was experiencing at the time. Her presentation was also seen to be in complete contrast with the way she had been described as acting for the past 40 years.

What triggered the supervisor's concern in the supervisory relationship was the resident's ambivalence in not pushing for the patient's immediate admission. By exploring the resident's ambivalence, and by framing it in a constructive manner, resident and supervisor were able to unravel the collusion of the family through denying the immediate risk of this patient with whom the urgency of the situation was not fully addressed (although even in hindsight a positive treatment plan was reached). It became clear, in fact, that the patient had been interviewed together with her daughters and husband, and their protective interference had masked the patient's powerful anxiety and projective identification. It only became clear later that the resident's family recently had his beloved grandmother admitted to a nursing home against her wishes because of her increasing senility, and he had felt guilty in not being able to prevent this decision. His passivity in this instance was a reflection of his guilt, as well as of the powerful denial and collusion evidenced within the family construct.

Are the identifications with patients in these situations counterproductive? This question centers mainly on the possibility that therapists may, by identifying with the person in need, react either by indulging them through a rescue fantasy, or by withholding and denying. Talbott (1980–1981) believes that what is much more common is an increased empathy and understanding in the therapist who is working with the patient in these situations than is the case in treatment of patients with many other psychiatric problems. The commonality of our shared experience of feelings engendered by the emergency/crisis situation supports our awareness that emergencies/crises are resolvable. Talbott points out that patients not only recover but can grow from the experience, and there are solutions to seemingly insolvable problems. He states—and I emphasize this point—that hospitalization may neither be a failure of crisis intervention nor an overresponse. It may in many instances represent the best form of emergency/crisis intervention. Communicating this position to residents is a very helpful and important experience in their psychiatric growth and education.

Summary

I have emphasized the psychodynamic perspective in the supervision of residents in providing an atmosphere in which the teaching and learning of emergency/crisis intervention can proceed. In so doing, I have used the psychodynamic life narrative, highlighted countertransference/transference positions in working with these patients, and illustrated the supervisory process between resident and supervisor. Clinical examples demonstrate the psychodynamic perspective that I believe can be useful and relevant for those who work in this area.

References

Bibring E: Psychoanalysis and the dynamic psychotherapies. J Am Psychoanal Assoc 2:745–768, 1954

Glick RA, Meyerson AT: The use of psychoanalytic concepts in crisis intervention. International Journal of Psychoanalytic Psychotherapy 8:171–188, 1980–1981

Greenacre P: On reconstruction. J Am Psychoanal Assoc 23:693–712, 1975

Harris N, Kalish B, Freeman E: Precipitating stress: an approach for therapy. Am J Psychother 17:471, 1963

Kahn A: The therapeutic stance, in Emergency Psychiatry: Concepts, Methods and Practices. Edited by Bassuk EL, Biric AW. New York, Plenum, 1984, pp 75–80

Stone L: Psychoanalysis and brief psychotherapy. Psychoanal Q 20:215, 1961

Talbott JA: Crisis intervention and psychoanalysis: compatible or antagonistic? International Journal of Psychoanalytic Psychotherapy 8:189–201, 1980–1981

Viederman M: The psychodynamic life narrative: a psychotherapeutic intervention useful in crisis situations. Psychiatry 46:236–246, 1983

Chapter 11

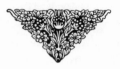

A Cognitive-Behavioral Model of Supervision With Individual and Group Components

Marsha M. Linehan, Ph.D., and
Debbie E. McGhee, B.A.

Graduate training programs in behavioral and cognitive therapies are widespread in clinical psychology. Cognitive behavior modification is ranked first (or tied for first) in training emphasis by two-thirds of clinical training directors in the United States (Nevid et al. 1986). Although behavioral and cognitive approaches have historically not been a substantive part of psychiatric training, their presence is increasing as the empirical bases of these approaches expand. Despite this prevalence, surprisingly few training or supervision models have been developed specifically for cognitive and/or behavioral approaches. Exceptions include a systematic model for behavioral supervision proposed by one of us (M.M.L.) in 1980, a social-learning approach developed by

Portions of this chapter originally appeared in Linehan MM: "Supervision of Behavior Therapy," in *Psychotherapy Supervision*. Edited by Hess AK. New York, Wiley, 1980, pp. 148–180. Copyright 1980 by John Wiley and Sons, Inc. Reprinted with permission.

Hosford and Barmann (1983), a multimodal supervision model developed by Ponterotto and Zander, and a collection of cognitive-behavioral techniques described by Kurpius and Morran (1988). What all of these models share is a supervisory focus on specific behaviors of the clinical supervisee (rather than presumed underlying dynamics), an emphasis on empiricism, and clear specification of the content and goals of therapy—characteristics that also describe behavior therapy in general.

The model of supervision we discuss in this chapter is a modification of the original model one of us developed (Linehan 1980). The modifications came about during the development and clinical trial of a cognitive-behavioral treatment (dialectical behavior therapy [DBT]) for severely dysfunctional, suicidal patients meeting criteria for borderline personality disorder (Linehan 1993a; 1993b; Linehan and Heard, in press; Linehan et al. 1991, in press). Borderline patients are notoriously difficult to treat even by the best of therapists. Their frequent suicidal and often angry behaviors create stresses that can derail individual therapists as well as entire treatment teams. Staff splitting, burnout and therapeutic mistakes, early dropout from treatment, and failed therapies are common with this population. Difficult patient populations are especially threatening within a clinical trial; the very behavior that brings these patients to therapy can interfere with their receiving the treatment the investigator wishes to evaluate.

Although a great deal has been written about training research psychotherapists for psychotherapy clinical trials, very little has been written about how to supervise research therapists so that they consistently provide therapy with a high level of skill. Facing these sorts of problems, the senior author of this chapter (M.M.L.) developed a model of treatment that in essence redefines psychotherapy as a system that includes treatment of the patient by a therapist or team as well as "treatment" of the therapist by a consultation-supervision team. Thus, from our perspective, supervision of therapists forms an integral part of treatment of patients. Although the model of treatment and of supervision was originally developed within a clinical research trial, the supervision methods have since been expanded to other clinical settings and now form an important part of our treatment program.

Goals of Supervision: Clinical Skills

Although almost everyone would agree that a principal goal of supervision is to help the supervisee become more effective in his or her clinical work, the specific skills needed to be effective are not always clear. At times the supervisee and supervisor may disagree on the relative importance of various treatment procedures and skills needed in general or in a particular case. In contrast to other forms of psychotherapy, cognitive and behavioral procedures and therapies are often manualized. When the focus of supervision is on teaching a specific treatment procedure, such as desensitization, or a manualized approach to therapy, such as Beck's (1976) cognitive therapy for depression, or Barlow and colleagues' (1989) behavioral treatment for anxiety disorders, a tension can develop between the need for flexibility on the one hand, and the need to learn how to apply a specified set of procedures on the other. When the therapy and supervision have been applied within a research context, this conflict must usually be resolved in favor of sticking with the research manual. Within nonresearch clinical settings, flexibility and creativity may win the day. From a behavioral supervisory point of view, however, both are equally important. Effective therapy requires clinical judgment, creativity, and flexibility, as well as skills in applying treatment interventions known to be effective even when the application is difficult or not self-evident.

Conflicts are especially likely to arise when the supervisee and supervisor disagree on the breadth of the goals. For example, a supervisor who believes the most important aspect of being an effective therapist is knowing and understanding oneself (e.g., Bergatino 1978) is likely to focus on broader objectives than those desired by a supervisee who views the goals of supervision as learning a narrow range of specified treatment techniques. The supervisee who wants to learn both a full range of effective procedures as well as skills of selecting, implementing, and evaluating treatments is likely to have trouble with the supervisor who is intent on teaching only procedures that have been labeled "behavioral" or who is only interested in teaching a very specific approach to therapy, such as one of the manualized treatments.

With these cautions in mind, it is still useful to outline those skills that must be developed if a person is to be an effective behavior therapist. Several lists have been generated (Collins et al. 1986; Lloyd and Whitehead 1976; Strosahl and Jacobson 1986; Sulzer-Axaroff et al. 1975; Thoresen 1972). Basing an approach on a tripartite model of human functioning, we have presented an extensive discussion of specific behavioral, emotional, and cognitive skills required of the behavior therapist (Linehan 1980). These skills are outlined in Table 11–1.

As can be seen, most of the skills outlined are generic and would be required of therapists practicing from any theoretical orientation. However, more so than most other treatment orientations, behavioral and cognitive therapies require a strong working knowledge of principles of and empirical findings on normal behavior. This is because behaviorists assume that "normal" and "abnormal" behaviors fall on a single continuum (i.e., the same behavioral principles apply both to adaptive as well as maladaptive behaviors [Kazdin 1978]). The behaviorist's insistence that therapists have a grasp of basic research on normal human functioning is similar to the general belief in medicine that to understand, diagnose, and treat disease, physicians must understand normal physical functioning.

Clinical supervision, in contrast to clinical training in general, assumes requisite knowledge. With beginning therapists and therapists who have not had extensive training in psychology, however, there is often an absence of this basic knowledge. For example, although psychiatric training covers the biological bases of normal and abnormal functioning, such programs rarely require residents to master principles of learning, empirical research on social-interpersonal behavior and influence, cognitive functioning, and so on. Thus, the psychiatric trainee in supervision can be counted on to have the requisite foundation in conceptual and empirical bases of pharmacotherapy; but the requisite knowledge base for psychosocial interventions, particularly empirical findings from experimental psychology, cannot always be counted on. In these cases, the behavioral supervisors may frequently need to assign extra readings or coursework to help the supervisee catch up and profit from the supervision.

Table 11–1. Goals of behavioral supervision: target areas and skills

System	Skill	Representative examples
Cognitive	Specific knowledge	Principles of normal behavior, including basic principles of learning, cognitive processes, and social and biological foundations of behavior
		Theory and research literature relevant to psychopathology
		Fundamental principles of behavioral theory
		Ethical and legal issues
		Research methodology
	Conceptual capabilities	*Ability to:* Organize and integrate information and apply basic knowledge of behavior to clinical problems
		Conceptualize cases and identify clinically relevant problems
		Plan effective treatment
		Make good clinical judgments
		Be aware of impact of one's own beliefs and values *and* those of the immediate and larger environments
Overt motor	Therapy-specific procedures	Assessment and treatment techniques
	Interpersonal-clinical skills	Communicate empathy, warmth
	Behavioral-clinical	Teach behavioral principles to client
	Professional	Engage in consultation, write reports
	Self-development	Outside reading, personal therapy
Physiological-affective	Control of problematic emotional responses	Monitor and manage reactions to the client (e.g., anxiety, anger, dislike)
		Monitor and manage reactions to the supervisor (e.g. evaluation anxiety)

Table 11–1. Goals of behavioral supervision: target areas and skills *(continued)*

System	Skill	Representative examples
	Attend to and manage arousal that is not emotion-linked	Self-monitor personal limits to avoid burnout

Behavioral Methods of Supervision: Strategies and Procedures

Clinical supervision requires skill in two somewhat antithetical tasks. On the one hand, the supervisor must find, value, and nurture the supervisee's inherent ability to help others in a clinically skillful manner. On the other hand, the supervisor must ascertain which skills are not in the supervisee's repertoire and assist the supervisee in acquiring these skills. The supervisor must step back and support natural development and autonomy while directing the supervisee's progress, confronting inadequacies, and influencing the supervisee's clinical work. Successful supervision requires the supervisor to weave together as whole cloth two sets of supervision strategies— problem solving and skills training on the one hand, and validation of existing supervisee responses on the other. The focus is on developing desirable skills in the supervisee (and eliminating clinically undesirable behaviors) while attending to and recognizing the truth in the supervisee's own experience. As in most clinical matters, the effective use of validation and skills training strategies requires sensitivity, astute timing, and flexibility to weave these two strategies together seamlessly.

Validation

One major function of supervision is to help the supervisee learn when to have confidence in his or her own judgment and natural responses to the patient. Validation strategies are useful in achieving this goal; they require the supervisor to search for and communicate the validity and wisdom in the supervisee's clinical work. Used effectively, validation in supervision consists of the same three steps we have described as essential to therapy (Linehan 1993a). Although these steps are at least implicit in all forms of supervision and are discussed intermittently throughout this chapter, it can be useful to gather them together to highlight their importance in the supervision process.

The first step is to listen to and observe the supervisee's clinical behaviors and to elicit his or her feelings, thoughts, and assumptions about the patient, the session under discussion, and so on. Behaviorists will generally emphasize the importance of the supervisor's actually observing therapy sessions, either live through a one-way mirror or on videotape. At a minimum, the supervisor should listen to tapes of the psychotherapy sessions.

The second step is to reflect back to the supervisee what is observed in a manner that the supervisee can understand. This requires that the supervisor let go of any preconceived ideas and actively observe what is happening. The emphasis here is on giving the supervisee feedback about what is actually observed rather than providing interpretations of the presumed meaning or underlying dynamics of the supervisee's behavior. Accurate feedback, in turn, requires that the supervisor let go of theoretical jargon when it interferes with being understood. The supervisor must also listen with a "third ear" to guess and test out any unstated thoughts, feelings, or beliefs that may be important in understanding the supervisee's clinical responses.

In the third step, after helping the supervisee observe and describe his or her emotional and cognitive experiences as well as clinical actions, the supervisor must search for and reflect back to the supervisee the wisdom or validity of the supervisee's clinical responses. The basic idea is that the supervisor must search for and find those areas of clinical judgment and action where the supervisee is responding in a clinically effective manner.

It is very important that validation not be confused with praise. Although praising a response that the supervisee also values is validating, praising a response that the supervisee believes was faulty or unskillful is invalidating—the supervisee learns to distrust rather than trust his or her own clinical judgment. For some supervisees, validating may require searching for the nugget of gold within a large cup of sand. For others, it may require only the merest polishing. In either case, it is essential that the supervisor consistently search for the "gold" and highlight it for the supervisee. Addressing the "cup of sand" is the function of problem-solving strategies we discuss later.

Cheerleading strategies are another form of validation and are the principal strategies for combating the supervisee's demoralization with especially difficult cases, or following particularly grievous clinical errors. In cheerleading, the supervisor communicates the belief that the supervisee is doing his or her best and validates the supervisee's ability to eventually develop therapeutic skills and provide effective treatment. It is not uncommon for therapists, especially those working with chronically suicidal patients, to feel that they are not doing anything worthwhile or helping their patients in the least. Here the supervisor may have to take out a magnifying glass to find and reflect the very small (but nonetheless hopeful) progress that the patient has actually made. Or it may require that the supervisor remind the supervisee that some approaches take time—lots of time. Overall, in cheerleading the supervisor expresses a belief in the supervisee, the patient, and the supervision relationship; offers reassurance; and highlights any evidence of progress. With new therapists and/or with very difficult cases, cheerleading may be the principal strategy of supervision.

Supervisory Problem Solving

Clinical supervisors must also assist the supervisee to assess and solve clinical problems he or she is faced with and to develop the skills necessary to implement solutions. When faced with nonskillful clinical responses or problems in the treatment being carried out by the supervisee, four primary questions must be addressed:

1. Does the supervisee have the requisite psychotherapy skills as described here? (For example, does the supervisee know what

procedures should be followed when intervening in a suicidal crisis?)

2. Is unskillful behavior due to faulty reinforcement contingencies within the therapy or the therapy training program (including supervision itself) such that ineffective behaviors of the supervisee are being reinforced, skillful behaviors punished, or rewarding outcomes delayed?

3. Is unskillful behavior due to a supervisee's pattern of avoidance within the therapeutic milieu, or are skillful therapeutic responses inhibited by unwarranted fears or guilt?

4. Is the therapist unaware of the contingencies operating within the therapy setting with this particular patient, or are skillful therapeutic responses inhibited by the supervisee's faulty beliefs or assumptions?

Depending on the answers to these questions, the supervisor may select from the various procedures described in the next section.

Skills Training

Skills training is an important part of almost all behavioral and cognitive approaches and forms an important part of behavioral supervision. Skills training procedures can be classified in terms of their desired functions (Rich and Schroeder 1976) and broken down into four categories: 1) response acquisition procedures, 2) response shaping and strengthening procedures, 3) response disinhibition procedures, and 4) response inhibition procedures (Linehan 1979). Although division of procedures into categories is, at times, arbitrary, it is useful to discuss each category separately. Detailed instructions on how to carry out each of the procedures are beyond the scope of our discussion. However, descriptions of the procedures can be found in many textbooks on behavior therapy (e.g., O'Leary and Wilson 1987) and cognitive-behavioral therapy (e.g., Beck and Freeman 1990) and are described in detail elsewhere (Linehan 1993a). What follows is a brief summary of some of the procedures used in behavioral supervision.

Response Acquisition Procedures

No matter how skilled the novice therapist, supervision will almost always involve the use of response acquisition procedures designed to teach the supervisees novel responses as well as new ways of patterning already existing repertoires. Response acquisition procedures include modeling of relevant skills and instructions. Modeling can be accomplished in a variety of ways. The supervisor can model directly by conducting therapy and engaging in other clinical activities the supervisee observes by one-way mirror or audio- or videotape, or by nonparticipatory sitting-in with the supervisor. In our training program for DBT as well as in many other behavioral treatment research clinics, for example, videotapes of the supervisor's own therapy sessions are readily available to all supervisees, and sessions with some patients can be observed through one-way mirrors. Supervisees are thus able to view the supervisor in action and to discuss the session in detail with the supervisor.

In addition, supervisors can model by describing clinical methods used in their own practices and how they accomplish other clinical activities, and by sharing their own values, beliefs, and conceptual models. Sharing of similar failure experiences, mistakes made, and unwanted emotional responses in the supervisor's own practice can be especially helpful in modeling how to cope with personal vulnerabilities and mistakes as a therapist. Group consultation (described in greater detail later) may often take the form of rap sessions in which the therapists (including the supervisor) share their thoughts on particular clinical issues and situations and how they might behave (or have behaved) when confronted with those issues in the therapy room.

Another powerful but often overlooked form of modeling that can be used in supervision is in vivo modeling. Here, the supervisor conducts him- or herself in a way that is consistent with (and reflective of) the therapeutic framework being taught. For example, DBT supervisors operate with their supervisees from within a dialectical framework, seeking to balance acceptance of the therapist where he or she is with a concomitant commitment to skill building (or change). Similarly, a supervisor may conduct a systematic behavioral analysis of the therapist's behavior with the patient in much the same way the therapist conducts behavioral analyses of the patient's actions. Thus, the behavior of the supervisor during supervisory sessions is directly parallel to his or her behavior with patients in therapy sessions. What in vivo modeling offers is the opportunity for the therapist-in-training to experience the methods of change at work. It would probably not be an overstatement to say that in vivo modeling is probably the primary instructional tool in the DBT framework.

Instructions can be given in any of a number of ways. Supervisees can be given books and articles to read; alternate methods of treatment can be suggested and discussed during supervision; the supervisor can teach some skills didactically; and on occasion, the therapist can be given direct instructions about how to proceed with a given case. While actively practicing their therapy skills, supervisees can be given suggestions through a "bug in the ear" device such that only they, and not the other person, can hear the supervisor (who is observing from behind a one-way mirror). Although this procedure is often used in actual therapy settings, especially in child and family therapy settings, it can also be used in structured training in role-playing. On occasion, if important decisions must be made immediately, the therapist can be instructed to leave the patient to consult with the supervisor before concluding the session.

Response Shaping and Strengthening Procedures

No matter what procedures are used, once the supervisee has acquired new responses, response shaping and strengthening procedures must be implemented to reinforce interpersonal and therapy skills that the supervisee already has in his or her behavioral repertoire and to ensure the development and stability of the new skills. Response shaping and strengthening procedures require practice of the relevant skills followed by feedback and reinforcement for skillful behavior and coaching for nonskillful behavior. Supervised clinical cases, of course, serve as a principal vehicle for shaping and strengthening skillful clinical responses. In the ideal case, the supervisee practices on the patient, and skillful behavior is reinforced by frequent and timely clinical improvement. Indeed, an important task of supervision is to teach the novice therapist to use patient feedback and progress as the primary response strengthening and shaping mechanism. Ultimately, it is the patient, more than the supervisor, who must direct the therapist's behavior.

When sufficient or timely reinforcement is not forthcoming from the patient, the validation strategies described here are the principal vehicle of supervisory reinforcement. Supervisory reinforcement is particularly important when the patient is providing immediate reinforcement for the therapist's behaviors that, in the long run, are iatrogenic or, conversely, if the patient is punishing therapist behaviors that ultimately would be effective. Such is often the case with borderline patients, for example, who frequently demand actions by the therapists that would either further reinforce their borderline behaviors (e.g., agreeing to wanted hospitalizations whenever the patient escalates crisis) or elicit conditioned maladaptive responses with which the patient cannot cope (e.g., demanding to talk about childhood abuse before the patient has even minimal skills to deal with the flood of emotions such discussions unleash).

Response Disinhibition Procedures

Response disinhibition procedures are designed to reduce or modify those factors that might be inhibiting the therapist from using skills that have been previously learned. Negative emotional responses can inhibit behaviors that would be helpful to the patient. For example, fears of closeness or personal exposure or excessive fears of violating "boundaries" can lead to stiffness and rigidity that interfere with the reciprocity necessary in clinical practice. In addition, unrealistic expectations and beliefs, or faulty application of values to the patient situation, can lead to the suppression of various clinically useful responses in which the therapist would otherwise be able to engage. The therapist who believes that patients will "fall apart" if verbally confronted is not likely to give critical feedback during sessions. Therapists who evaluate persons with problematic behavior patterns as "sick, pathological manipulators," or who use other value-laden and pejorative terms, are not likely to either respect their patients or assess and use the patients' strengths.

A therapist who believes that if a therapist cannot do effective therapy he or she is not a good person (or must have difficulty relating to people, or can never help anyone) is likely to be so concerned with negative evaluations that he or she has trouble thinking clearly during sessions. A therapist who expects to never dislike patients, never feel angry, never feel sexually aroused by or attracted to a patient, never feel threatened by a patient, never feel nervous, and so on, is likely to mislabel such feelings and thus not use them when they might be informative in the treatment sessions. Dodge (1982) has noted that evaluation anxiety can interfere with the learning process within supervision itself and recommends that supervisors employ cognitive-behavioral techniques to help supervisees alleviate such anxiety.

It is also important to closely examine the supervisory relationship and the therapist's training program for factors that may be inhibiting useful clinical behaviors. For example, the supervisor may be inadvertently punishing the supervisee for using procedures that do not fit the supervisor's theoretical position but that nonetheless would be quite effective if tried. Or the supervisor may confuse "style" with "strategy" and criticize stylistic approaches natural to the supervisee that do not fit the supervisor's view of effective clinical behavior. Training programs often inadvertently set up expectations for clinical behaviors that, while generally effective, interfere with clinical effectiveness in specific cases. The ability to examine the environment for factors that inhibit effectiveness, either by reinforcing ineffective behavior or by punishing effective clinical behaviors, is itself an important clinical skill. Therefore, such examinations, when carried out within the supervision process itself, have the added benefit of modeling how to go about this task.

A number of procedures can be used to facilitate response disinhibition. The most common procedure in behavioral supervision, as in other forms of supervision, is to combine a continuing dialogue about the therapist's own values, beliefs, and goals with supervisory modeling of the desired (but inhibited) responses. On occasion, as noted by Levine and Tilker (1974), the supervisor may need to use verbal confrontation as a procedure for helping the supervisee attain more realistic labeling of his or her values and beliefs, and their possible consequent effects on clinical behavior. One helpful procedure is peer-group discussion of clinical experiences. Often the very sharing of fears and concerns is useful in alleviating them. In difficult cases, the supervisor might employ a more structured approach, combining desensitization, shaping, and reinforcement of approximations of the desired clinical responses. In other cases, referral to personal therapy may be necessary so that the supervisee can work on issues interfering with his or her work.

Response Inhibition Procedures

Response inhibition or suppression procedures are used when the goal is to stop iatrogenic clinical responses occurring in therapy. When and how frequently these procedures should be used depend on a number of factors. With new supervisees, where inhibition related to anxiety is already so great, much more emphasis will be put on response disinhibition and reinforcement of skillful responses already in the supervisee's repertoire. With more experienced therapists, therapists in supervision as a result of serious difficulties delivering competent or ethical therapy, or therapists trying to replace one approach to treatment with another (as is often the case in training experienced therapists for clinical trials), the supervisor may give more critical feedback and rely more on confrontation of problematic therapist responses.

In each case, inappropriate therapy responses made by the supervisee must be replaced by more useful responses. Punishment (i.e., any aversive procedure, including criticism, confrontation, expression of dismay, etc.) must be used with caution and balanced carefully with the validating strategies described here. Most often, rather than punishing the old response, the supervisor can just as easily suggest or otherwise teach new responses to take its place.

The superiority of reinforcement over punishment techniques in teaching behavioral skills is well documented (Feldman and Broadhurst 1976). An important side effect of punishment or aversive techniques is that they frequently increase supervisee anxiety. High anxiety can in turn both interfere with new learning and disrupt the trainee's own natural clinical responses.

A second common side effect of punishment is to make the person delivering the punishment less potent as a source of future reinforcement. Thus, when punishment is used in supervision, interpersonal distance arises between supervisor and supervisee. This distance and decreased potency as a reinforcer have a range of negative effects, including decreasing effectiveness of the supervisor as a teacher. Furthermore, the negative effects on the relationship between the therapist and the supervisor that punishment often carries with it can trickle down and affect the relationship between the therapist and the patient. If a therapist is anxious and fearful of his or her supervisor or wants nothing more than to be rid of that supervisor, it is likely that less learning will take place and/or the therapist will be less enthusiastic about the case in general. In the end, it is the patient who suffers most in such a situation.

Models of Supervision

As we have noted, clinical supervision can be carried out individually or in groups. All of the strategies discussed so far apply to both modes. A peer-group supervision mode has been developed that is designed originally for treatment of severely dysfunctional and suicidal patients who meet criteria for borderline personality disorder (Linehan 1993a). The procedures, however, are applicable to supervision of any hard-to-treat clinical population. A number of caveats about supervision groups based on the Linehan model are in order. First, as we have noted, this mode does not differentiate supervision from therapy itself. Therapy is defined as the treatment of a community of patients by a community of therapists where the welfare and change in the patient is guided directly by one or more of the therapists (in group and individual psychotherapy) who are in turn "treated" by the supervision-consultation team (in individual or group settings). It is this ongoing transaction among patient, therapist, and supervision team that accomplishes the therapeutic work. Thus, supervision in the Linehan treatment approach is necessary for *all* therapists, novices and experts alike.

Second, the "treatment of the therapist" (i.e., the supervision process) is the application of the same treatment procedures to the therapist that the therapist applies to the patient—only the behavioral targets differ. With patients, the focus is on reducing maladaptive responding (i.e., behavior, emotions, cognitions) in their everyday lives and replacing these responses with more adaptive and satisfying ones. In supervision, the context of focus is strictly limited to the clinical situation. That is, the "treatment" of the therapist is restricted to enhancing the therapist's clinical skill and actions. The supervision model is based on DBT, and balancing or synthesis of dialectical tensions is viewed as essential to the supervision as it is to the therapy.

There are three functions of a supervision group in the Linehan approach. First, the group is the system within which the treatment is developed and implemented. Cases are presented and discussed, and all group members actively work to generate solutions to problems in treatment. Furthermore, group members are available for consultation with each other between group sessions when the need arises. With suicidal patients, availability of the training supervisor is particularly important. In this capacity, the group provides feedback and coaching. Second, the group cheerleads, moralizes, and remoralizes the therapist whenever necessary. The group holds the therapist's hand behind the scene, so to speak, keeping the therapist within the therapeutic relationship and frame. In this capacity, the group reinforces effective behaviors, even when patients are providing immediate punishment for those very same behaviors. Third, the group balances the therapist in his or her interactions with the patient. The group highlights the oppositions inherent in the therapist's position, asks "what is being left out" of the therapist's position, and encourages a dialectical stance on the part of the therapist. The most fundamental dialectic is that between acceptance (of self, the patient, the team, and the therapeutic relationship and rate of progress) on the one hand and change (of perspective, treatment methods, understanding of the patient, and interactions with the team) on the other.

Within this dialectical supervision framework, a number of principles apply. First, it is expected that all therapists will attend weekly supervision group sessions, whether or not they also receive individual supervision. The group is designed in a peer supervision format, wherein each member shares case material from the preceding week. Second, it is expected that all therapists will abide by a set of guidelines that, taken together, organize the type of group interactions. The guidelines apply to all members of the group, including the training supervisor, who may be the official leader of the group. Although the guidelines were originally written for guiding DBT, they can be generalized to other treatment approaches as follows.

Accepting a Dialectical Philosophy

First, the supervision group agrees to accept, at least pragmatically, a dialectical philosophy. When polarities arise, the task is to search for the synthesis rather than for absolute truth in any one position. The dialectical agreement does not proscribe strong opinions, nor does it suggest that polarities are undesirable. Rather, it points to the direction therapists agree to take when polar positions that are passionately held arise.

Elsewhere, we have listed a number of polarities likely to arise in therapy (Linehan 1993a). The most fundamental, as we noted previously, is that between an orientation of acceptance versus that of change. Others likely to surface in behavior therapy include the tension between giving and wanting autonomy versus taking control and wanting directions; a deterministic position versus one that suggests personal responsibility and free will; and a view of behavior as operant (i.e., controlled by its consequences) versus classically conditioned (i.e., controlled by eliciting stimuli). These polarities are no less likely in supervision, both as tensions within supervision itself and as a problem to be solved within therapy. Strongly felt polarities are especially likely to arise in at least two situations: when the patient is very difficult to treat and when the therapy being proposed or offered is nontraditional, at least in the terms of the supervisory group. With difficult patients, a common polarity is between the "let's get tough" attitude and the "patient-is-fragile" attitude. When new or unorthodox treatments or therapeutic stances are the issues, the polarity may revolve around that of safety and legal cover for the therapist and supervisors versus creativity and possibly more effective treatment. Over time, each individual's position on the polarity is likely to fluctuate, even for the same patient.

Such polarities are often the precipitants of splitting—between supervisor and supervisee, therapist and supervision group, and/or therapist and patient. The prior agreement by members of the supervision group to seek synthesis by searching for the truth in both sides of arising polarities can be extremely effective in short-circuiting further conflict. In our experience, the simple fact of a prearranged rule of conduct seems to be a critical factor in allowing individuals with very intensely held beliefs to relax their hold long enough to move toward resolution. In a group setting, where the rule of dialectical resolution is clear, all members of the group are expected to actively call for and search for synthesis.

Observing Personal Limits
When Conducting Therapy

The supervision group then agrees that all therapists are to observe their *own* limits when conducting therapy. "Limits" in this sense refers both to personal limits of doing therapy and limits of effectiveness (i.e., those imposed by what is necessary for clinical progress in a particular case). The goal is to make sure that the contingencies operating in therapy do not punish the therapist's continued involvement. The Linehan strategy of "observing limits" was developed to replace the usual practice of "setting limits" proposed by many therapy manuals. The position taken is that therapists must take responsibility for monitoring their own personal and professional limits and clearly communicate to patients which behaviors are tolerable and which are not. When treating difficult patients, therapists who do not do this will eventually burn out, terminate therapy, or otherwise harm the patient.

Because natural limits are favored over arbitrary ones, the limits will vary between therapists and with the same therapist over time and circumstance. However, observing one's own limits is much more difficult than following a list of arbitrary limits written in a book or given by a supervisor. With novice therapists, in particular, simply knowing personal limits can be extremely difficult. As one therapist said in our group, it is impossible to know some limits before they are crossed. Indeed, a fundamental goal of all supervision, in general, is to assist therapists in discovering their own personal limits as therapists and in learning which professional behaviors cross the limits of effective treatment. Group members agree not to judge other therapists' broad or narrow personal limits. Serious problems with limits, however, are dealt with individually by the training supervisor.

Accepting the Fallibility of Therapists

Group members also agree a priori that all therapists (including experienced training supervisors) are fallible. Mistakes not only will be made, but may be made repeatedly with difficult patient populations, and often with not-so-difficult patients. The position taken in our group supervision meetings is that most mistakes patients accuse us of making we probably have made. We have observed that even very experienced and ordinarily good therapists often do bad therapy with suicidal and borderline patients. This observation was the principal force behind the development of the supervision-consultation team mode of treatment (Linehan 1993a). However, the idea *here* is not that all therapists are doing "bad" or ineffective therapy. Rather, it is that all good therapists make mistakes. An essential component of many good therapies is the effective repair of therapeutic errors.

In essence, this agreement is a commitment to be nondefensive at the start. As a norm set at the beginning, it says to each member of the supervisory group that "perfection" is not expected, that errors are not catastrophes, and that clinical skill is going to be found in how well a therapist admits to mistakes and proceeds to repair them, not necessarily (within reason) how well they are avoided in the first place. The team acknowledges the "tear in the therapeutic fabric" and assists the therapist in figuring out how to mend it therapeutically. The task of the supervision team is to apply the problem-solving strategies described here to help each other improve in clinical effectiveness. As with patients, however, problem solving with therapists must be balanced with validation of the inherent understandability of the therapist's stance. Because, in principle, all therapists are fallible, group members all agree that they will inevitably violate all of the agreements at times, including all those listed here. When this is done, supervision group members rely on each other to point out the polarity and move to search for synthesis. Very serious therapeutic errors will usually also need to be discussed in individual supervision.

Helping Each Other Understand and Conceptualize Patient Behavior

As in all supervision groups, an additional task of group members is to help each other understand and conceptualize patient behavior in a theoretically consistent manner. An important aspect of cognitive-behavioral therapy, of course, is helping the therapist conceptualize the case in behavioral and/or cognitive terms and develop treatment plans consistent with the theoretical understanding. In our supervisory groups, team members are also charged with assisting therapists in conceptualizing patient behavior in ways that reduce the therapist's tendencies to maintain a hostile attitude or push the patient away (on the one hand) or to develop excessive sympathy, unrealistically low expectations, and overnurture the patient (on the other). It is not unusual in our groups for a therapist to walk in and say "I'm furious and I'm going to kick my patient's butt! Help me find another way to think about this" or on another occasion to say "I'm furious at everyone who is being bad to my patient, and I'm going to pull her out of every environment where people aren't sufficiently sympathetic to her terrible pain! Give me another way to think." The supervisory team's task is to do just that—to help the therapist synthesize his or her current position with a position representing the "other side of the story."

In many settings such as clinics and inpatient units, more than one therapist interacts with the same patients. In these settings, staff splitting and consequent splitting of the treatment team and supervision group is especially likely. From our point of view, at least, these interactions form an important component of the overall treatment system (Linehan 1993a). The next two guidelines were developed to ameliorate problems in this area and to guide staff interactions so that a therapeutic frame could be maintained. Because these supervision guidelines have more to do with how therapy itself rather than how supervision per se is conducted, the guidelines are mentioned but not elaborated upon.

Avoiding the Role of Intermediary

Therapists agree to avoid the role of intermediary for patients with other members of the supervision team. Thus, when therapists behave fallibly (within reason), the task of each of the other therapists on the supervision team is to help patients cope with the therapist's behavior, not necessarily to reform the therapist. Treatment problems and planning are discussed in a consultative rather than authoritative manner.

Agreeing to Accept Diversity

Finally, the supervision team agrees that consistency of therapists with each other is not necessarily expected. Each therapist does not have to approach the patient similarly or teach the same thing, nor do all have to communicate the same rules. Each therapist can make his or her own rules about conditions of the therapeutic relationship with the patient. Diversity is respected rather than abhorred.

Conclusion

We have attempted to set forth the essence of a cognitive-behavioral model for supervision developed out of our work with severely dysfunctional patients meeting criteria for borderline personality disorder. In DBT, supervision is one of the core components of the therapeutic system, required of both novice and experienced therapists. A number of principles underlie this model.

First, in DBT supervision, as in all cognitive-behavioral models in general, the focus is on identifiable behaviors of the supervisee, rather than on underlying dynamics. Thus, the supervisor directs his or her attention to overt behaviors, cognitions, and/or emotional responses that influence the supervisee's work with the patient.

Second, all behavior is seen as lying along a continuum from normal to abnormal, rather than perceiving normal behavior as being somehow fundamentally different from abnormal behavior. Thus, the same behavior-change principles that are used to facilitate change in the patient can be applied in supervision to facilitate change in the therapist. We have set forth what those strategies and procedures are insofar as they relate to supervision.

Third, the characterization of psychotherapy is broadened to include not only the patient/therapist dyad but also the therapist/supervisor relationship. In other words, therapy is seen as a *system* in which the supervisor (or supervisory team) works to modify or control the behavior of the therapist. The goal is to make therapist behavior consistent with the therapeutic model and in the best interest of the patient (and the therapeutic relationship), while the therapist works to modify the behavior of the patient in a direction that is more adaptive and functional.

Finally, acceptance versus change is the key dialectic that guides the supervisor's (or consultation team's) work. The challenge is to successfully balance validation of the supervisee's experience and actions with an insistence on modification (or change) of his or her behavior, in a direction that is theoretically consistent and maximally therapeutic.

References

Barlow DH, Craske MG, Cerny JA, et al: Behavioral treatment of panic disorder. Behav Res Ther 20:261–282, 1989

Beck AT: Cognitive Therapy and the Emotional Disorders. New York, International Universities Press, 1976

Beck AT, Freeman A: Cognitive Therapy of Personality Disorders. New York, Guilford, 1990

Bergatino L: A theory of imperfection. Counselor Education and Supervision 17:286–292, 1978

Collins FL, Foster SL, Berler ES: Clinical training issues for behavioral psychology. Professional Psychology: Research and Practice 17:301–307, 1986

Dodge J: Reducing supervisee anxiety: a cognitive-behavioral approach. Counselor Education and Supervision 21:55–60, 1982

Feldman MP, Broadhurst A: Theoretical and Experimental Bases of the Behavior Therapies. London, Wiley, 1976

Hosford RE, Barmann B: A social learning approach to counselor supervision. Counseling Psychologist 11:51–58, 1983

Kazdin AE: History of Behavior Modification: Experimental Foundations of Contemporary Research. Baltimore, MD, University Park Press, 1978

Kurpius DJ, Morran DK: Cognitive-behavioral techniques and interventions for application in counselor supervision. Counselor Education and Supervision 27:368–376, 1988

Levine FM, Tilker HA: A behavior modification approach to supervision of psychotherapy. Psychotherapy: Theory, Research and Practice 11:182–188, 1974

Linehan MM: A structured cognitive behavioral treatment of assertion problems, in Cognitive Behavioral Interventions: Theory, Research and Procedures. Edited by Kendall PC, Hollon SD. New York, Academic Press, 1979, pp 205–240

Linehan MM: Supervision of behavior therapy, in Psychotherapy Supervision. Edited by Hess AK. New York, Wiley, 1980, pp 148–180

Linehan MM: Cognitive Behavioral Treatment of Borderline Personality Disorder. New York, Guilford, 1993a

Linehan MM: The Skills Training Manual for Treating Borderline Personality Disorder. New York, Guilford, 1993b

Linehan MM, Heard HL: Impact of treatment accessibility on clinical course of parasuicidal patients: in reply to R.E. Hoffman [letter to the editor]. Arch Gen Psychiatry (in press)

Linehan MM, Armstrong HE, Suarez A, et al: Cognitive-behavioral treatment of chronically parasuicidal borderline patients. Arch Gen Psychiatry 48:1060–1064, 1991

Linehan MM, Heard HL, Armstrong HE: Naturalistic follow-up of a behavioral treatment for chronically suicidal borderline patients. Arch Gen Psychiatry (in press)

Lloyd ME, Whitehead JS: Development and evaluation of behaviorally taught practice, in Teaching Behavior Modification. Edited by Yen S, McIntire RW. Kalamazoo, MI, Behaviordelia, 1976

Nevid JS, Lavi B, Primavera LH: Cluster analysis of training orientations in clinical psychology. Professional Psychology: Research and Practice 17:367–370, 1986

O'Leary KD, Wilson GT: Behavior Therapy: Application and Outcome. Englewood Cliffs, NJ, Prentice-Hall, 1987

Rich AR, Schroeder HE: Research issues in assertiveness training. Psychol Bull 83:1081–1096, 1976

Strosahl K, Jacobson NS: Training and supervision of behavior therapists. Clinical Supervisor 4:183–206, 1986

Sulzer-Axaroff B, Thaw J, Thomas C: Behavioral competencies for the evaluation of behavior modifiers, in Issues in Evaluating Behavior Modification. Edited by Wood WS. Champaign, IL, Research Press, 1975

Thoresen CE: Training behavioral counselors, in Implementing Behavioral Programs for Schools and Clinics. Edited by Clark FW, Evans DR, Hamerlynek LA. Champaign, IL, Research Press, 1972

Chapter 12

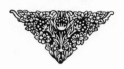

The Development of a Psychotherapy Supervisor

Leopoldo Chagoya, M.D., F.R.C.P.C, and
Charlotte Chagoya, R.N, PG Psych. Nurs.,
Dip.Fam.Ther.

Our theoretical framework in this chapter is psychoanalytic, integrating object relations, intersubjective, and interpersonal systems theory concepts. We focus on the development of the supervisor of individual psychotherapy, although some of our concepts apply to the teaching of other forms of psychotherapy.

"I feel like a fraud," a female resident in supervision said.

"You are," answered the male supervisor—partly seeking a paradoxical effect, partly trying to desensitize the resident to a taboo subject. The somewhat aggressive comment served to elaborate on a truth that pertains to all practitioners and supervisors.

"We all begin as frauds," he continued. "That is the nature of

We gratefully acknowledge the cooperation and the editorial comments of Drs. Stanley E. Greben and Ronald Ruskin, and the generous sharing of ideas by Drs. Joel Sadavoy, Daniel Silver, Rodney Slonim, and Graeme Taylor.

the learning of psychotherapy. As we read, apply theories and techniques, and learn the vicissitudes of the patient-therapist-supervisor interaction, we grow to be less and less fraudulent, and eventually mature into the real thing."

The beginning of a career as a supervisor can be a fortuitous event. The budding teacher is invited to supervise by the more experienced ones, or finds him- or herself supervising others by virtue of having attended courses or workshops not available to colleagues. At times, after a clinician shows a videotape of his or her work or presents a clinical demonstration or a paper that seems practical and applicable, someone in the audience privately asks to be supervised by the presenter. In any case, once a clinician is engaged in a teaching career, supervision becomes an inevitable and expected didactic activity.

History

Balint (1948) mentioned that Freud did not like to supervise. Neither he nor Ferenczi, Abraham, or Jones included supervising as an important activity in their curricula. Only when the Berlin Institute of Psychoanalysis was established in 1920 was the supervision model of teaching formalized. Betcher and Zinberg (1988) describe how, early in the psychoanalytic movement, Hungarian and Viennese schools of supervision developed. The Hungarians maintained that a control or training analysis was of utmost importance, because it would effectively serve as supervision, as it would deal with the therapist's irrational feelings about the patient. The Viennese Psychoanalytic Institute, on the other hand, maintained that the student's personal analyst should not supervise the student's first cases and that different points of view should be presented by the supervision, in the hands of someone other than the personal analyst of the candidate.

Grotjahn (1955) reports that in the 1920s and 1930s, few papers were published expressing concern about the supervision phenomenon. Yet from the 1950s on, symposia on supervision became a common occurrence, headed by psychoanalytic authorities like Sloane (1957), Kubie (1958) and Ekstein (1960). In 1965, the *Collected*

Papers of Searles included his articles "The Informational Value of the Supervisor's Emotional Experiences," and "Problems of Psychoanalytic Supervision." In 1970, the *International Journal of Psycho-Analysis* included several papers exclusively about supervision.

Some authors have criticized supervision as a process that goes against the basic psychoanalytic principles of free association and self-observation, precisely because it demands that the supervisee take notes and remember. As Kubie (1958) remarked,

> [We] ask [the student] to be free and bound in the same moment of human interchange, to react freely, to participate in a complex emotional interchange with his patient, to observe, to take notes, and to tell objectively how a session proceeded. This means we are asking the candidate to do something impossible. The best the student can do is leap back and forth from one [function] to the other. (p. 229)

Kubie concluded that it is a miracle that supervision is useful at all.

Freud wrote about psychoanalytic education in "The Question of Lay Analysis" (1926/1959) and in the "New Introductory Lectures on Psychoanalysis" (1933/1964). Yet he did not examine the process of supervision.

Psychoanalytically oriented supervision usually emphasizes intrapsychic dynamics and intersubjective factors between patient and therapist (Greben 1991). The teaching of other approaches has emphasized interaction, cognition, behavior, or other premises and objectives.

Objectives

As the supervisor matures, he or she changes his or her objectives in the teaching endeavor. At first, his or her method may be tinged with narcissistic overtones, as the supervisor may try to show the student his or her skill, knowledge, and accuracy. In time, the supervisor slowly realizes that the educational process has to be collaborative and must take into account the personality, preparation, and style of the supervisee, who usually wants to succeed.

The supervisor has to define if he or she will treat the patient through the student (which defines the apprentice as a mere carrier of interpretations), or if he or she will partially relinquish (as long as it is safe) the responsibility for the patient and pay attention strictly to what the supervisee does, both during the session with the patient and during the supervisory session.

Wolberg (1967) defines the following as functions for supervision: 1) to help the student develop a "psychotherapeutic" instrument; 2) to make a pedagogic diagnosis of the obstacles the student finds in his or her learning; 3) to give the supervisee didactic objectives related to the effect of his or her own behavior on the patient; and 4) to help the supervisee examine his or her relationship with the supervisor.

As the supervisor learns the craft, he or she shapes personal answers to many questions.

1. How authoritarian or directive will he or she have to be with students at different levels of expertise?
2. Will it be sufficient to ask searching questions to redirect the attention of the supervisee?
3. Will it be useful to say: "At this point I would intervene and remark on . . . ?"
4. Will it be necessary to suggest directly that the supervisee employ a certain technique, still leaving him or her the freedom not to use it?
5. Will it be essential to pressure the supervisee to do something with the patient even if the student is not convinced of the value of that intervention, or to stop doing something that may be deleterious for the patient or for the supervisee?
6. Will it be necessary to approach the boundaries of psychotherapy for the supervisee (Rubin 1989) and point out countertransferential or personal conflicts that interfere with the therapy process or with the supervision process?

Paraphrasing some of Freud's comments on education (1933/1964), we may apply them to some aspects of psychotherapy supervision. According to Freud, the superego, as it develops, receives also the influence of the persons that take the place of the parents: the educators, the teachers, and the persons the individual chooses as ideal models. The identifications with these late parental beings contribute in an important manner to the formation of the character, but in this case they affect the formation of the ego, not of the superego, which was determined by earlier parental images (p. 64). The child has to learn to control his or her instincts; therefore education must inhibit, prohibit, and suppress, to find the adequate balance between the noninterference and the frustration. It is a matter of deciding how much to forbid, when, and through which means. Children have different dispositions; therefore, the same educational process can not possibly serve for everyone. The task of the educator is to recognize the individuality of the child and to give him or her the adequate amount of love, maintaining nevertheless an effective degree of authority (pp. 149–150).

However, supervisors have to temper these statements and not apply them verbatim to the supervisee. He or she is an adult who therefore requires from the supervisor a manifest adequate respect for his or her stage of ego maturation.

Supervision may give the supervisee a therapeutic experience when it produces a psychological stress that activates personal conflicts (Wadder-Hall and Sloane, quoted by DeBell 1963). The student uncovers factors of his or her personality that are an obstacle to contact with the patient, sees where the gaps are in his or her theoretical knowledge, realizes when a certain type of intervention is opportune and when it is not, and decides whether the patient he or she chose for supervision is appropriate (Chagoya 1978, 1981).

The supervisor may create a difficulty for the student by demanding that he or she find a patient with a specific defense constellation. If the clinical population available to the student does not include the type of individual the supervisor wants, the supervisee's enthusiasm could be undermined by the exigencies of the supervisor. It seems preferable to accept any patient the student is interested in, to start as soon as possible, and to use the process of supervision to help the supervisee ascertain whether the patient is suitable or not. We can compare this process with learning how to use a photographic camera. The target focused is not that important; mastering the instrument is.

Remus considers the supervisor an auxiliary ego who helps the student integrate his or her experiences with the patient (A. J. Remus, personal communication, Mexican Psychoanalytic Association, November 1978). Arlow (1963) adds that the supervisor must observe the vicissitudes and the pathology in the capacity to be empathic with the patient, and then confront the student with reality by giving him or her information and examples of the supervisor's own experience. Arlow does not consider supervision to be an adequate method to help the supervisee solve unconscious conflicts. But Tamez (1963), using his own experience, maintains that adequate interventions by the supervisor can solve paralyzing unconscious conflicts. Fleming and Benedek (1964) assert that the alliance to learn between supervisor and supervisee is similar to the therapeutic alliance between therapist and patient.

The usual supervisory activities include the following:

1. Focusing the student's attention on the blind spots of his or her understanding of the patient (transference and dynamics);
2. Pointing out the interventions (or the silences) determined by the student's countertransference as well as the effect of the student's behavior on the patient;
3. Providing for the student clinical examples of successful or failed interventions, taken from the supervisor's practice; and
4. Commenting, when necessary, on the type of relationship the student establishes with the supervisor.

Sachs (1947) wished to help the student maintain a strong scientific skepticism, recommending that supervisors not allow the student to see him- or herself as a descendant of Prometheus, who will bring the light to those who walk in darkness, lest "the student feels as an extremely shortsighted leader of the blind" (p. 168).

The supervisor has to be empathic toward the patient and toward the student, analyzing a therapeutic process, not the student as an individual. Bibring (quoted by Grotjahn 1955) believed that the center of supervision is advice, not personal interpretations nor commands. Catalytic questions or comments may promote insight in the student. The supervisor may see him- or herself sometimes as the patient's therapist. At other times, the supervisor's self-perception may be as an observer of what happens inside the student—how the student relates to and communicates with the patient, how much the student can observe him- or herself, and to what degree he or she is in contact with personal, preconscious motivations. At all times, the supervisor has to be aware of the relationship with the student in the here and now and observe how he or she responds during the supervisory hour (Greben 1976, 1979a, 1979b).

Technique

The technique of supervising varies from one teacher to another. Some demand a written version of the session. Others discourage this method because when a session is read, intellectualization increases and affect is inhibited. Nevertheless, as the supervisor learns to pay attention to the intonation the student uses to recount the session, he or she will perceive the countertransferential affect and use it as supervision material. Kubie (1958) believed that the student who reports more details is perhaps the least perceptive and least faithful to the sessions described. Countertransferential material is also spontaneously revealed in stammering, pauses, asides, and in what the student emphasizes or minimizes. At times, the supervisor can observe how a student hides behind a written version of the session and is incapable of reconstructing fluently the affective flow of his or her contact with the patient. Taking notes during the session decreases the free-floating attention of supervisees and may distract them from analyzable unconscious material. In "Recommendations to Physicians Practicing Psychoanalysis," Freud (1912/1958) underlines the convenience of listening before anything else, without worrying whether or not it will later be possible to remember something about the session. He reminds us that the bigger the effort a person makes to attend to or note something specific in the session, the more he or she selects and loses sight of other areas, following personal inclinations or expectations. In view of all this, the supervisor has to be interested also in the "unconscious memory" of the candidate.

When all goes well, students gradually increase their self-confidence and their affective and unconscious contact with the patient. It is noticeable then that supervisees need their notes less and less to reconstruct the session. There comes a time when the supervisory hour is not enough to present all the material the student remembers; in the initial phases of supervision, he or she could only fill a few minutes while strictly reading his or her notes. Peltz (M. Peltz, personal communication, May 1979) supervised while he and the student walked; other teachers supervise using audiotapes (Harmatz 1975; Kubie 1958) or videotapes (Chodoff 1972) of the session. The supervisor may observe students supervising each other, or use role-playing to illustrate transferential and countertransferential issues (i.e., one student recreates the session and another plays the role of the patient, with immediate feedback [Ekstein 1960]).

Grotjahn (1955) described a situation where supervisees are asked to listen in while a colleague is supervised, or where the supervisor shares a session with a student and the patient. In doing this, the supervisor may talk to the patient as if he or she were a cotherapist, or may take over completely as a consultant, or even talk exclusively to the student about the patient or about the session's process. If the supervisor chooses this latter technique, he or she has to politely reject any attempt by the patient to engage him or her in a dialogue.

Betcher and Zinberg (1988) have maintained that supervision through audiotaping, videotaping, or observing the therapy sessions through a one-way mirror invades the privacy of the therapist and the therapy. This intrusion, they believe, increases the self-consciousness of the therapist and modifies the character of the therapy. Betcher and colleagues plead for granting a certain amount of privacy to the therapist as an essential ingredient of effective supervision.

Characteristics of the Supervisor

The characteristics of the supervisor that influence the process are as follows:

1. Personality and character, degree of maturity, and amount of unresolved neurotic conflicts;
2. Theoretical background;
3. Technical preferences;
4. Ease in communicating affectively and effectively in a didactic manner with the supervisee; and
5. Type of relationship the supervisor establishes with the supervisee.

The supervisor may address the student as a colleague. But if neurotic elements prevail, he or she may treat the supervisee as a son or daughter (idealized or devalued), as an inferior, as a menacing presence who will show the supervisor's shortcomings to a higher authority, or as another type of transference figure.

The supervisor gradually learns that personal expectations about teaching reflect his or her own libidinal investment in the supervisory task. He or she also understands, little by little, which are his or her defensive reactions when the student resists, devalues, or avoids learning.

At times, the administrative structure of the institution where the supervisor and the supervisee interact may affect the process of supervision. This may happen, for instance, by imposing a certain supervisor on a student or vice versa, by not giving the supervisor the supportive environment he or she requires, or by politically undermining the efforts of the supervisor. As a supervisor develops, he or she learns to recognize these factors and tackles them directly, thus fostering a free flow of interaction with the student.

In some institutions, when the supervisor belongs to a professional group different from that of the young therapist, interdisciplinary politics may complicate the development of trust and respect in both directions. For instance, a medical resident may find it hard to accept a social worker, a psychologist, or a psychiatric nurse-therapist as his or her supervisor in psychotherapy. By the same token, a nonmedical supervisor may use the teaching situation to redress hierarchical tensions in the way he or she treats the student. It is the supervisor's task to maintain and promote interdisciplinary respect and confidence.

Research

Shanfield and colleagues have devised and researched the reliability of a scale to rate supervisors' behaviors (Shanfield and Gil 1985; Shanfield et al. 1989). Studying videotaped supervisory sessions, these investigators measure seven content scales (focus on the therapist, focus on the patient, intellectual orientation, experiential orientation, number of clarifying and interpretive comments, intensity of confrontation, and depth of exploration), and six interaction scales (verbal activity level of the supervisor, dominance of the supervisor, dominance of the therapist, comfort level, tension level, and empathy of the supervisor). In a form devised at Mount Sinai Hospital to evaluate clinician-teachers for the University of Toronto, students rate their supervisor's level of knowledge, ability to communicate, relevance to students, punctuality, availability, enthusiasm, overall level of ability as a teacher in the Faculty of Medicine, and overall level of ability as a teacher in the Department of Psychiatry.

Perez and colleagues (1984) studied residents' perceptions of the teaching of psychotherapy in Canadian psychiatric residency programs. The supervisor's profile that the subjects favored included capacity to develop a good rapport with trainees, teaching ability, ability to pinpoint the resident's psychotherapeutic shortcomings, and willingness to help residents overcome them. The subjects in this study also pointed out that insufficient attention was given by psychotherapy supervisors to formulating treatment approach and goals, and to practicing techniques of transferring patients to another therapist and terminating therapy.

At the Family Court Clinic of The University of Toronto, H. McDonough and J. Steadman (personal communication, March 1992) are investigating the usefulness of an evaluation form for supervisors that estimates the number of hours of supervision, observed interviews, and reading assignments; kinds of feedback given to the student about his or her progress; enthusiasm, organization, clarity, and level of knowledge; direct clinical demonstrations of skills by the supervisor; and amount of modeling he or she provides for the supervisee.

Intrapsychic and Transference-Like Factors

When positive affect predominates in the teacher, he or she will approach students with patience and benevolence and criticize with tact, taking care to not wound the supervisee's narcissism too much. Reider (quoted by Ekstein 1960) believed that the supervisor's interventions should be seen as hypotheses for the supervisee to test, not as orders to obey. The positive teacher invites the student to review what he or she has done, does not devalue the session (which is a fait accompli), and helps the supervisee recognize when factors in his or her personality originate countertransference obstacles. Here the supervisor may stride the fine line between supervision and personal psychotherapy for the student. In any case, genetic interpretations should never be part of a supervisory process.

The student may represent for the supervisor a son or daughter he or she wishes to see grow. Yet a narcissistic investment of the educator in the student is constructive only if it does not stop him or her from pointing out the mistakes or the conflicts of the young therapist. If the teacher limits him- or herself to a kind of seduction of the student through open or subliminal praise, he or she does not help the student's growth. Support of the student, though necessary, is not enough. Furthermore, if the student and the supervisor join too closely, they may share blind spots about the patient.

The adequate supervisor learns to think with his or her student. He or she openly talks about being perplexed at certain moments of the treatment and keeps in check his or her own omnipotent tendencies and those of the student. Because he or she tolerates narcissistic wounds, the supervisor welcomes the questioning of suggestions made and the growing autonomy of the supervisee.

At the other end of the spectrum, when the transferential components in the supervisor are predominantly negative, he or she may be subtly persecutory, threatening, challenging, or ridiculing. The supervisor may overload the novice with references and insist that the student be successful with untreatable patients, which maintains an atmosphere of threat in the supervision. The young therapist may represent for the neurotic supervisor an Oedipal rival child he or she wishes to destroy, or a child object of jealousy because he or she has more freedom than the supervisor ever had when he or she was in training. The supervisor may then feel he or she should apply to the supervisee the rigor of times long gone. At times, through displacement as a defense mechanism, conflicts between two supervisors may affect the way each teacher approaches the student.

The supervisee's personality may elicit affection, irritation, or intimidation in the supervisor. A kind of rivalry may appear between teacher and student (probably an interplay of projective identifications). If this occurs, the supervisor may show impatience, disdain, tentativeness, indecision, lack of interest, or sullenness during the supervision. At times, he or she may give the student the sensation that therapeutic ability is an intangible abstraction that cannot be taught.

The supervisor may act out with the supervisee a protest against administrative or professional authorities. This may show in how long the supervision session lasts (too much or too little), in how punctual the supervisor is, or in the content of the supervisory sessions. DeBell (1963) states that the teacher can use the supervision to satisfy his or her own narcissism and undertake the search for disciples as if to form a cult, promoting the identification and dependence of the students and falling into dogmatism. The discerning kind of students that populate teaching institutions in the 1990s usually reject this kind of teacher.

The supervisor caught in a negative relationship with the supervisee may show subtle condescension or hostility. Such a supevisor may infantilize the candidate, resent the supervisee's progress or minimize his or her successes, produce dominance/submission fights, or (as a reaction formation against his or her own aggressivity) become oversolicitous and excessively friendly.

At times, the institutional grapevine or formal reports about the supervisee's previous performance may create positive or negative expectations in the supervisor. The teacher has the task of not ignoring previous reports, but not allowing these ideas to blind him or her to the student's traits that contradict, positively or negatively, what other supervisors have seen.

Other chapters of this book deal with how differences in gender or cultural backgrounds between supervisor and supervisee affect the supervision. It is part of the supervisor's development to be conscious of these factors and integrate them in his or her teaching technique.

Status and Roles

In the supervisory situation, one of two people wishes to assume the position of educator, and the other the position of learner. One wishes to teach and the other to receive the teaching. One defines him- or herself as expert, the other as an apprentice. If the two complementary roles are well defined and accepted, the process will flow without difficulty. However, if this does not take place—if one of the two does not accept that, in the hierarchy that is necessarily there, one has more and one has less psychotherapeutic experience—there may be conflict.

At times, the supervision does not proceed unless the *supervisor* accepts putting him- or herself in the role of the learner. However, in other situations, the supervisor has to grasp how to deal with the student who does not accept the learner's position, whether because of interpersonal dynamics or because the supervisor belongs to a discipline that administratively is not at the top of the institutional hierarchy. Sometimes the student had belonged to a higher administrative level in previous positions and finds it hard to accept a kind of demotion, even if essential to learning new psychotherapeutic skills. The supervisor then has to contain the vicissitudes of the supervisee's loss of status.

As the supervisor becomes seasoned, he or she understands how to cope with the student who will come to supervision to prove that there is nothing the instructor can teach him or her, or who will seek supervision only to confirm a frozen ideology (Wolberg 1967) or to try to indoctrinate the supervisor with ideas not in keeping with the supervisor's specialty. In these predicaments, the teacher may have to confront the student—not interpreting at a genetic level (i.e., not making reference to the student's family of origin), but commenting at an interactional level on the obstacles that have appeared in the teaching/learning process.

Keissler (quoted by Sloane 1957) advised allowing the young therapist to fail, so he or she will realize he or she has to do something to change the situation. However, this advice seems risky in light of the patient's welfare.

Because of conflicts about status, the supervisor may decline to assume the expert position or embrace the loneliness of the educator. He or she may declare that the supervisory role is "only as a colleague who will learn with the student" and avoid exercising authority or using personal experience. The supervisor may thus cause the student to think: "If this person does not have a lot to teach me, as he or she humbly declares, what am I here for?"

Communication

The student-teacher dyad exchanges verbal and nonverbal messages—conscious and unconscious comments about the treatment of a patient, the hierarchical position of each member of the dyad, the relationship that both have with the administrative institution that to an extent controls them, and a philosophy of psychotherapy and an existential philosophy. Yet the supervisee or the supervisor may not have the ability to communicate didactic material to each other. The student may understand his or her patient much better than he or she is able to convey to the supervisor and may distort the therapy sessions to the extreme of presenting "another patient"; or the supervisor may be so cryptic or abstract that the student remains unsupervised.

Dissolution of the Dyad

Most training programs impose a time limit on the contact between supervisor and student. They separate at the end of the academic year, regardless of the level of expertise the young therapist has achieved. It is part of the teaching/learning experience to prepare the student for the end of the supervision, to establish a countdown of the final sessions, and to gear their content around aspects of separation, mourning, individuation, and autonomy. The supervisor has to deal with his or her own feelings and to find a way to let the supervisee go, even if the supervisee is not quite well formed yet. A positive process of supervision ends with mutual respect and gratefulness for the reciprocal teaching both members of the dyad have received.

In the case of a negative process of supervision, sometimes a kind of divorce has to be implemented. The antagonistic supervisor-supervisee dyad has to separate when mutual trust and respect cannot be developed despite a reasonable effort made by both members. If there is too much acting-out behavior in the student, the teacher, or both, they have to examine what happened, probably with the help of colleagues or in personal psychotherapy, so as not to repeat the situation with new students or new supervisors.

When supervising is no longer rewarding for the teacher, it is time to consider a change of activity and to review why the enthusiasm, essential for successful supervision, is missing.

Training for Supervisors

Who teaches the supervisor how to supervise?

Being a good therapist does not mean being an adequate supervisor. Meetings, seminars, and interconsultations among supervisors and supervision of the supervision help (Frayn 1991). Martin and colleagues (1978) have recommended an open dialogue among students and teachers about the process and problems of supervision, so all can examine why certain supervisors are popular and others unpopular. Issues of shame, fear of hurting the pride of colleagues, and political issues may inhibit discussions about who is or is not an adequate supervisor, and about why this is so.

Feder has mentioned that, given that the supervisor is transferentially a kind of lover/parent/mentor, he or she learns this métier by having many children, and by trying not to repeat with subsequent offspring the mistakes he or she made with the first ones (L. Feder, personal communication, Western Regional Psychoanalytic Societies

Meeting, Los Angeles, CA, May 1979). DeBell (1963) believed that the majority of supervisors intuitively reach their own functional style of teaching.

Aronson has asserted that every supervisor has his or her own theory of therapy, whether it has been explicitly formulated or not (G. Aronson, personal communication, Western Regional Psychoanalytic Societies Meeting, Los Angeles, CA, May 1979). Such theory includes objectives, techniques, elements deemed inadmissible, favored elements, and rationales to support conventional or nonconventional ways of giving therapy. The supervisor conveys all this to the supervisee through words, gestures, mood, and silence during certain moments of the supervision. Teacher and student develop, accommodate to each other (Shanfield et al. 1989), and formulate and test the theory of therapy that the supervisee proposes. The dyad must increase the education and maturation of both. The young therapist has to develop his or her own style, and the supervisor has to mature his or her own style of teaching.

According to Lindon, supervision reaches its goal when it is maturational and therapeutic for both the supervisee and the supervisor, whereupon both increase their insights and their unconscious receptivity (A. Lindon, personal communication, Western Psychoanalytic Societies Meeting, Los Angeles, CA, May 1979).

To end this chapter, we summarize the answers from six experienced supervisors in response to four specific questions on their development as psychotherapy supervisors. Our colleagues are S. E. Greben, R. Ruskin, J. Sadavoy, D. Silver, R. Slonim, and G. Taylor from the Department of Psychiatry at Mount Sinai Hospital in Toronto.

▼ How did you become a psychotherapy supervisor?

It was not planned. Because I was always interested in psychotherapy and in supervising, I was asked to do it, first with medical students and interns and then with residents.

I wanted to follow the model of the emotionally accessible teachers I experienced.

▼ What has been the most useful idea for you in your development as a supervisor?

The concept that there are numerous ways in which the psychotherapist can use him- or herself to treat patients. The supervisory process is best when it brings out the innate ability of the therapist to find his or her own best path to manage patients.

Supervision is collaborative. Two people work together to understand.

Teaching a mind-set that helps the supervisee to see what is going on between him or her and the patient and, for me, acquiring a mind-set that helps me to see what is going on between me and the student, and between the students and their patients.

Being able to put myself in the shoes of the residents, and through empathy understand their struggle, their wonder, their curiosity to learn how to become better at what they do, and also their anxiety and concern about being judged or criticized.

Learning to not have the same expectations from every resident, but to adapt them to his or her level of knowledge and sophistication. I have to adapt my style to teach pretty basic things when it is necessary.

▼ What has been the most difficult problem in your development as a supervisor?

To tolerate not knowing how to help the student, which reflects the ambiguity of therapy.

Becoming comfortable with the pressure to be the expert in the early stages of supervision.

Dealing with unsophisticated or defensive students, who are so concrete they cannot comprehend the abstract ideas necessary for psychotherapy. Some are not interested in it; the residency program compels them to do it. We have to help these residents to come to an honest self-evaluation, because not every one of them should do psychotherapy.

Motivating and maintaining a teaching alliance with residents who resist in the form of not finding suitable cases for supervision. Some residents have engaged in a form of splitting, devaluating me as unreasonably hard for expecting them to find a case, complaining about me to the Director of the Department, and idealizing another supervisor. As this process has been worked through, it has been reversed.

To help students who are extremely defensive to deal with serious countertransference issues, which become an impediment to therapy. Some are unwilling or unable to discuss impediments to psychotherapy that stem from their morality or their sexual orientation. They feel they cannot introduce these issues in the supervision, because they are unable to respond to the empathy of the supervisor.

To teach residents with little theoretical background who therefore do not have the awareness necessary to plan a therapeutic strategy or conceptualize what is happening to the patient.

Deciding when to teach theory during the supervisory process.

To keep silent and let the therapist find his or her own way through the process of supervision.

Guiding without imposing a rigid formal structure, because learning psychotherapy is a self-generated guided process.

To decide when or how to grade the didactic process.

The misconceptions about psychotherapy some supervisees bring with them and the repeated attempts the supervisor has to make to bring the supervisee around to abandon such misconceptions.

Dealing with my own vulnerabilities as a person and exposing those vulnerabilities to the supervisee.

Turning around the aversion a resident seemed to have toward me.

Differentiating between the supervision of psychotherapy and the supervision of psychoanalysis.

How to gently, kindly, and humanely encourage residents with no talent for psychotherapy to look at interesting alternatives in psychiatry, so that psychotherapy becomes a minor part of their work. I do not believe we can teach every resident psychother-apy. Some are more talented than others for it. For some, all we can teach is part of the basics, or an attitude, but often we do not discourage them from doing psychotherapy.

▼ How do you think psychotherapy supervisors should be trained?

By using the knowledge available from educational research and from specialists in methods of teaching.

By doing supervision, by reading what sensible authors have written about it, and by sharing ideas with other supervisors, so we learn from each other's clinical experiences in supervising.

By acquiring a sense of oneself through personal psychotherapy or psychoanalysis, experiencing what it is like to be a patient.

By listening carefully to what the residents have to say about the supervisor.

By having a great deal of supervision from experienced super-visors with different theoretical perspectives, so that I can, from the exposure to a wide range of theoretical perspectives, synthe-size my own perspective.

The supervisor and the supervisee undertake an investigative jour-ney during which both learn from each other. Besides what we have already mentioned, in order not to stagnate and to keep their skills sharp, supervisors have to participate in discussions at diverse edu-cational centers, where other supervisors review their work. This exposure allows teachers to renew their methods and consider ideas that may be absent from their usual circle. That way, learning continues for psychotherapy supervisors as long as they practice their art.

References

Arlow JA: The supervisory situation. J Am Psychoanal Assoc 2:576–594, 1963

Balint M: On the psychoanalytic training system. Int J Psychoanal 29:163–173, 1948

Betcher RW, Zinberg NE: Supervision and privacy in psychotherapy training. Am J Psychiatry 145:796–803, 1988

Chagoya L: Clinical supervision in the field of child psychiatry [in Spanish], in Monografías de la Asociación Mexicana de Psiquiatría Infantil. Num 3, México, DF, 1978

Chagoya L: On the process of supervision [in Spanish]. Cuadernos de Psicoanálisis 19:40–64, 1981

Chodoff P: Supervision of psychotherapy with videotape: pros and cons. Am J Psychiatry 128:819–823, 1972

DeBell D: A critical digest of the literature on psychoanalytic supervision. J Am Psychoanal Assoc 11:546–575, 1963

Ekstein R: Report of the panel on the teaching of psychoanalytic technique. J Am Psychoanal Assoc 8:167–174, 1960

Fleming J, Benedek T: Supervision: a method of teaching psychoanalysis. Psychiatr Q 33:71–96, 1964

Frayn DH: Supervising the supervisors: the evolution of a psychotherapy supervisors' group. Am J Psychother 45:31–42, 1991

Freud S: Recommendations to physicians practicing psychoanalysis (1912), in The Standard Edition of the Complete Psychological Works of Sigmund Freud, Vol 12. Translated and edited by Strachey J. London, Hogarth Press, 1958, pp 113–114

Freud S: The question of lay analysis (1926), in The Standard Edition of the Complete Psychological Works of Sigmund Freud, Vol 20. Translated and edited by Strachey J. London, Hogarth Press, 1959, pp 183–250

Freud S: New introductory lectures on psychoanalysis (1933), in The Standard Edition of the Complete Psychological Works of Sigmund Freud, Vol 22. Translated and edited by Strachey J. London, Hogarth Press, 1964, pp 64, 149–150

Greben SE: Supervision of psychotherapy with psychiatric residents: one model. Canadian Psychiatric Association Journal 21:141–144, 1976

Greben SE: The influence of the supervision of psychotherapy upon being therapeutic, I: introduction and background to the supervisory relationship. Can J Psychiatry 24:499–506, 1979a

Greben SE: The influence of the supervision of psychotherapy upon being therapeutic, II: modes of influence of the supervisory relationship. Can J Psychiatry 24:507–513, 1979b

Greben SE: Interpersonal aspects of the supervision of individual psychotherapy. Am J Psychother 45:306–316, 1991

Grotjahn M: Problems and techniques of supervision. Psychiatry 18:9–15, 1955

Harmatz MG: Two-channel recording in the supervision of psychotherapy. Professional Psychologist 6:478–480, 1975

Kubie LS: Research in the process of supervision in psychoanalysis. Psychoanal Q 27:226–236, 1958

Martin GC, Myerson P, Olson HE, Wibers LL: Candidates' evaluation of psychoanalytic supervision. J Am Psychoanal Assoc 26:407–424, 1978

Perez EL, Krul LE, Kapoor RK: The teaching of psychotherapy in Canadian psychiatric residency programs: residents' perceptions. Can J Psychiatry 29:658–664, 1984

Rubin SS: At the border of supervision: critical moments in psychotherapists' development. Am J Psychother 43:387–397, 1989

Sachs H: Observations of a training analyst. Psychoanal Q 16:157–168, 1947

Searles HF: Collected Papers on Schizophrenia and Related Subjects. New York, International Universities Press, 1965

Shanfield SB, Gil D: Styles of psychotherapy supervision. Journal of Psychiatric Education 9:225–232, 1985

Shanfield SB, Mohl PC, Matthews K, et al: A reliability assessment of the psychotherapy supervisory inventory. Am J Psychiatry 146:1447–1450, 1989

Sloane P: Reports on the second panel on the technique of supervised analysis. J Am Psychoanal Assoc 5:539–545, 1957

Tamez GR: An account of transferential and countertransferential chain reactions [in Spanish], in Psicoanálsis, La Técnica, Monografías Psicoanalíticas 9. Edited by Palacios A, Ramirez S, Valner G. México, D.F., Asociación Psicoanalítica Mexicana, AC, Editorial Pax., 1963, pp 192–201

Wolberg LR: Supervision of the therapeutic process, in The Technique of Psychotherapy, Part 2. New York, Grune & Stratton, 1967, pp 1027–1054

Chapter 13

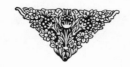

Privacy Versus Disclosure in Psychotherapy Supervision

Elizabeth Wallace, M.D., F.R.C.P.C., and
Anne Alonso, Ph.D.

Exploring and sharing self-experience are integral components of human relationships. The relationship between a trainee learning the complex art and science of psychotherapy and an experienced psychotherapist as teacher has at its center the teaching, modeling, and repeating of some aspects of the psychotherapist's experience of being with a patient. As the supervisory relationship develops and unfolds, there evolves a dynamic tension and interplay between the dual pulls toward privacy on the one hand and disclosure on the other with respect to the trainee's experiences in learning psychotherapy.

The pull toward disclosure on the part of the trainee is fueled not only by the wish for connection with an admired teacher, who may come to serve as an object for identification, but also by the necessity of exposing psychotherapeutic work in order to learn (Alonso 1985). Supervision is based on the premise that the trainee will disclose (as fully as possible) what has occurred in the interaction between trainee-therapist and patient, and in addition, will discuss feelings that are pertinent to the interaction. The mandate for the trainee may be stated as: "Say what occurred; present what you do, but also share your conceptual perspective of what you are presenting; reveal all, including the experience of your own participation" (Bromberg 1984). This mandate to disclose is reminiscent of what is asked of the patient in psychotherapy or psychoanalysis, dating from Freud's explication of the fundamental rule: "Never forget that you have promised to be absolutely honest and never leave anything out because, for some reason or other, it is unpleasant to tell it" (Freud 1913/1958, p. 135).

Adequate disclosure is essential to supervision, because the supervisor depends on information provided by the trainee to broaden and deepen understanding of the patient and to foster development of the trainee's psychotherapeutic skills. Omission of significant information about the therapy, in the form of "secrets" on the part of the trainee, can and often does lead to diminished clinical effectiveness and loss of key learning opportunities that occur through exposing mistakes as well as "hidden" strengths. (We discuss some exceptions later in this chapter.)

The assumption that the trainee in fact tells the supervisor most events and feelings related to the psychotherapy experience is not always borne out in practice. Research and literature about psychotherapy education have not addressed the issue of privacy versus disclosure in depth, although many authors refer to the importance of both issues in supervision. One author has noted that some psychoanalytic candidates confess to falsifying material or censoring data in supervision, based on fear of their supervisors' evaluation (Chrzanowski 1984). Supervisees experience conflict in choosing between presenting what makes them look good, and what makes them look bad—the latter being where help is usually most needed (Greenberg 1980). Students may also tend to omit discussion of their own participation and reactions, instead focusing on the behavior of the patient and thus maintaining an emotional distance from the material (Issacharoff 1984). Conscious and deliberate distortion of process notes may occur, with editing out of material which is deemed likely to provoke criticism from a particular supervisor (Betcher and Zinberg 1988).

These observations concur with our experiences as trainee and supervisor (supported by discussions with psychotherapy students at various levels of training) that students more or less consciously omit discussion of significant information about their psychotherapy experience to varying degrees, at different stages of training, with reference to certain psychotherapy patients and issues, and in relation to different supervisors.

The pull toward privacy in supervision occurs at several levels. At an intrapsychic level, privacy represents an inner space needed to work through painful affects associated with mistakes, narcissistic injuries, or other difficult experiences that happen when working intensively with patients (Brightman 1984–1985). The same inner space provides an arena for sexual feelings and fantasies to be safely explored. Privacy is also needed for the development of autonomy. At an interpersonal level, the experience of supervision, although necessary for learning, can be viewed as a personal intrusion that produces anxiety. Trainees in supervision may be even more anxious than patients in therapy, because trainees lack a clear center for presenting themselves in relation to the psychotherapy material, which deprives them of certain defenses. In fact, the ambiguity around supervision can leave all parties to the process confused and alarmed, especially when the patient seems to be getting sicker or not to be progressing.

In talking about interactions with patients, trainees inadvertently reveal a great deal about their own personalities. Both patients in therapy and trainees in supervision may need to defensively modify their stories. Privacy can thus be viewed as essential for supervision as well as to development of an individual therapist's style (Betcher and Zinberg 1988). At a social systems level, psychotherapy and psychoanalysis are social forms that exist in a culture of secrecy, where supervision represents a "leak" in the system (Rustin 1985). Trainees may at times feel torn between their duty to keep their patients' secrets confidential, and their own need for education that requires disclosing secrets in supervision.

Several processes must be distinguished that may alter the trainee's report about his or her psychotherapy experiences. The first involves the largely unconscious process by which interchanges with the patient, or related feelings in the therapist, are forgotten or modified. We might argue that all people must arrange conscious truths about themselves in a manner that is syntonic enough to be borne by the ego under stress. Such alteration is a function both of the nature of the therapy process (which, like dreams, quickly escapes recall) and a function of the therapist's defensiveness (Betcher and Zinberg 1988).

The supervisory process places the trainee in the impossible position of being expected to accurately describe to an observer the details of an event in which the trainee was involved as a participant. The reconstruction of a therapy session necessarily involves the selection of perceptions (Bromberg 1984). Supervisors may or may not be aware of such alterations in the material presented by trainees, but they may choose to implement recording devices or direct observation in an attempt to increase the accuracy of material available for supervision.

Comparing the discrepancy between process notes and recordings of sessions raises the question of the importance of authenticity versus accuracy in supervision (Betcher, quoted in Zinberg 1985). A second process, which is the focus of this chapter, concerns the conscious or at least partly conscious omission or alteration of material by the trainee for purposes of supervision. The latter process may operate even with recording devices or observation, if the trainee shifts the process of alteration from supervision into the interaction with the patient. In addition, discussion of the trainee's feelings and thoughts—an important source of information for supervision—relies on self-report, not observation. A serious learning problem may arise if the trainee begins to mute his or her fantasies or associations about the work to stay safe in supervision. The inability to express these feelings and fantasies, of course, puts the student at greater risk of acting on them.

When deciding whether or not to expose certain events or feelings in supervision, the trainee has three conscious options: to disclose the material to the full extent of his or her awareness; to disclose the material in part by selectively omitting or modifying details, or altering the context of the material; or to omit the material entirely from discussion. We conceptualize privacy and disclosure as existing on a continuum, with the balance of tension shifting in either direction on the continuum at a given point in time during supervision. At the far end of the privacy spectrum is the trainee of dubious renown in many training programs, who is rumored to have fabricated ongoing psychotherapy sessions for the purpose of supervision, neglecting to disclose that the patient has dropped out of treatment. At the other extreme of disclosure is the trainee who feels compelled to reveal details of therapy and personal feelings to such an extent that supervisory boundaries become blurred, the supervisor is overwhelmed, and learning and integration are blocked. Most supervisory interaction likely falls between these extremes on the privacy/disclosure continuum. The following case example illustrates the situation of two trainees working in this "middle zone" in supervision, somewhere between privacy and disclosure.

> A resident was beginning her third year of residency in psychiatry at a new setting located very far from her previous rotation. She planned to continue intensive psychotherapy with her long-term psychotherapy patient during the new 6-month rotation, because during the initial year of therapy they had established a good therapeutic alliance and transference manifestations had begun to develop. After several weeks, the patient noted that although she felt very much in need of ongoing therapy, she could not manage the long trip from her workplace and was in danger of being fired. The resident was sympathetic, as she had experienced similar difficulties traveling to the new location and did not wish to terminate the therapy, because of the patient's level of distress and her own educational needs.
>
> The resident had just met her new psychotherapy supervisor. Without discussing her dilemma, the resident arranged to see the patient at a borrowed office—one that was more centrally located—at the end of the day. Although both patient and therapist felt that this was a reasonable alternative in the short term, the resident avoided telling her new supervisor, expecting that he would view her actions as overly gratifying to the patient. Several of her previous supervisors had suggested that she was too accommodating and flexible with respect to patients' scheduling requests, thus avoiding underlying factors of resistance and transference.

To the resident's surprise, after a brief period of calm in the new office, the patient became angry and hostile toward her. The patient could not verbalize what had triggered her sudden change in attitude, and the resident was mystified as to why her previously grateful patient was now so devaluing. She felt increasing anger toward the patient, who no longer seemed to appreciate her doctor's accommodation to her needs. The resident felt guilty that she may have made a terrible mistake.

As she got to know her new supervisor, she revealed more about the psychotherapy sessions and sought help in understanding her patient's hostility. However, she did not mention the change in location of sessions and edited out any revealing material when presenting her process notes. The supervision was thus of limited help to the resident in understanding the patient's and her own anger and confusion.

The resident mentioned her dilemma to a friend in fourth-year residency. The fellow resident recalled that she had arranged to see a long-term psychotherapy patient in an alternative setting after an incident during her rotation on a chronic psychiatric inpatient unit. While waiting for an appointment with the doctor, her patient had been harassed by a psychotic inpatient on the ward and had vowed never to return to the hospital. The resident felt guilty, as the patient had already accompanied her to three settings during training, and she thus offered to meet with the patient at another office. Although she felt that the decision had a positive effect on the therapy, she never told her supervisor about the change. Her supervisor had previously commented that the resident's psychotherapy patients would "just have to get used to" being seen at the chronic inpatient setting, and she did not want to disappoint her supervisor by revealing her divergent views. That resident had had a warm relationship with this supervisor for several years, as evidenced by their final supervisory session during which she gave her supervisor a gift and burst into tears.

The first resident, feeling supported by her colleague's experience, decided to present the truth to her supervisor in an altered time frame. She now told him that the patient was angry because of the increased transit time to sessions and subsequent threats from her workplace; this situation had in fact existed several months previously. She presented her idea about borrowing a more central office (in fact a fait accompli) and though her supervisor was somewhat surprised and dubious, he did not oppose the plan. She then proceeded to close the time gap between what was occurring in psychotherapy and what she presented in supervision. When she revealed the patient's initial gratitude about the change of location followed by hostility, the supervisor helped the resident to examine what her actions may have meant to the patient. The patient admitted that she felt tremendous guilt and pressure to change after the move, in return for her therapist's accommodating behavior. She resented this greatly as it reminded her of her mother's martyr-like behavior. The supervision was now of great value in understanding the transference and countertransference issues involved.

This case example illustrates nondisclosure in two different supervisory contexts. The first resident had not yet established a trusting alliance with her supervisor and chose to keep an important decision about the therapy secret until the supervisory relationship had further developed. The second resident, in contrast, omitted significant information well into the relationship with a highly valued (and perhaps idealized) supervisor whom she did not wish to disappoint. In terms of level of training, both were senior residents who had developed some skill as psychotherapists and were comfortable in making some autonomous decisions about their patients. Disclosure and privacy are thus influenced not only by the developmental stage of the trainee but also by the developmental stage of the trainee-supervisor relationship.

Theoretical and Developmental Underpinnings

The trainee's decision to disclose information or to maintain privacy in supervision may be understood from several developmental and theoretical perspectives. Such perspectives are relevant, because the novice trainee-therapist progresses through various developmental stages in the course of forming and consolidating a professional self during training. These stages are reminiscent in some respects of the process of child and adolescent development. Areas to be considered here include narcissism and shame, autonomy and identity formation, and development of self and intersubjectivity.

Narcissism and Shame

The trainee-therapist occupies a position of narcissistic vulnerability on several counts. Acquisition of new psychotherapy skills involves a learning regression in which professional self-esteem is threatened by exposure of therapeutic work to an idealized other who possesses knowledge and skills available to the trainee only through experience (Alonso and Rutan 1988a). The fledgling therapist's performance is unlikely to measure up to his or her professional ego ideal for some time, and thus the trainee's sense of self-esteem is shaky.

Kohut (1971) describes a transitional period in development on the way to mature narcissism characterized by the grandiose self and the idealized parent imago. The trainee's grandiose professional self is buffeted by the experiences of not knowing enough and not feeling in control of the clinical work. At the same time, the supervisor is required to serve as an idealized supportive figure with whom the trainee can ally him- or herself. Disclosure of problematic material in psychotherapy supervision can pose threats to both the grandiose self (which may experience deflation and humiliation) and the maintenance of the relationship with the idealized other, if the trainee fears that disclosure will result in loss of the supervisor's admiration and respect. A significant amount of energy may be invested in concealing the image of the professional self as ignorant, destructive, and helpless (Brightman 1984–1985), which impinges significantly on the trainee's degree of sharing with the supervisor.

Shame is a painful affect frequently mentioned by trainees when describing reasons for nondisclosure in supervision. Shame has been understood differently by various theoretical schools. For example, object relations theory links shame to the loss of the object and thus basic unlovableness (Blatt 1974), whereas self psychology emphasizes disintegrative anxiety, which produces shame related to empathic failure (Morrison 1986). Shame can be experienced by the person alone as a negative judgment about the self, or later in development as humiliation in relation to more powerful others (Alonso and Rutan 1988b). Shame has a powerful impact on the trainee's level of disclosure in supervision, particularly for shame-prone individuals who cannot move beyond the privacy of their painful affects, even in the presence of a sympathetic supervisor. Shame is a particularly potent inhibitor of trainee disclosure regarding sexual and aggressive feelings in the psychotherapy encounter. We present some examples later.

Autonomy and Identity Formation

The trainee's movement between privacy and disclosure dovetails with the developmental process of separation-individuation and identity formation as a psychotherapist. This process has been described as the trainee "trying on a series of borrowed and patched vestments" (VanBuskirk 1969). In other words, the repeated process of imitation, identification, and introjection of aspects of the supervisor occurs over the course of learning psychotherapy. This process may result in incorporation of the introjects into the student's personal and professional identity or, alternatively, separation and ejection from the ego (Ford 1963). This process recurs during the course of training as the student moves toward consolidation of a professional identity.

At certain points in learning, the trainee has greater needs for closeness with and assistance from the supervisor, which may be manifested by increased disclosure and dependency-like requests for the supervisor's involvement. In counterpoint are the trainee's movements toward separation, which involve the trainee's experiments with new formulations and interpretations before consultation with the supervisor. Autonomy requires periods of privacy in which the trainee's thoughts and actions are played out in the psychotherapeutic arena with minimal intervention on the part of the supervisor.

The trainee's growth of autonomy in the relationship with the supervisor is illustrative of Mahler's description of the practicing subphase of separation-individuation, which highlights the growth of autonomy in close proximity to the mother (Mahler et al. 1975). The major achievement of upright locomotion heralds the first unaided steps, which are usually in the direction *away* from the mother or in the mother's absence. The mother's confidence in the child's practicing steps is an important trigger for the child's feeling of safety and pleasure in autonomy. The psychotherapy supervisor must allow for the trainee's practicing steps in doing psychotherapy while remaining encouraging and in proximity. Optimal supervision fosters the trainee's capacity to be alone in the presence of another, and to maintain mutuality in the course of separation.

Just as too much disclosure on the part of the trainee may signal an overly dependent relationship with the supervisor, too much privacy may indicate premature autonomous development. Adolescent experiments with danger are often premature experiments with autonomy preceding development of adequate self-regulation and judgment. Trainees may borrow and flirt with novel therapeutic techniques that they have observed or read about, without adequate knowledge of the potential impact on their patients. The supervisor, analogous to a parent, plays a role in setting limits on the trainee's activity with patients, with requests for more disclosure as needed. On the other hand, the supervisor needs to tolerate risk taking and appropriate levels of danger so that the trainee may gain enough confidence and learn his or her own limits, and to do this while there is still the built-in opportunity for supervision of the work.

Intersubjectivity and Development of Self

Disclosure about the psychotherapy experience during supervision invariably involves some degree of self-disclosure on the part of the trainee-therapist. The greater the exposure of "self" in the material, the greater the anxiety involved in disclosure, and the more likely that "secrets" will develop. Self-exposure is experienced most intensely when trainees describe their own behaviors, interventions, and counterreactions with respect to their patients. Thus, supervisors are frequently nonplussed to find that abundant material related to the patient contrasts with a paucity of descriptive information about the trainee's contribution to the interaction.

The literature pertaining to self-disclosure has focused primarily on the experience of the patient in psychotherapy. However, some parallels can be drawn to the situation of the trainee in supervision. Disclosure of self is an intersubjective process that requires a receiver as well as a transmitter (Josephs 1990). Self-disclosure serves dual functions. It is an interpersonal act of communication that promotes intimacy; intrapsychically, however, it is also a vehicle for enhancing self-definition through listening to self-perceptions that are stated out loud.

In psychotherapy supervision, a degree of self-disclosure by the trainee is essential to convey information to the supervisor. The process serves as a substrate for learning about such issues as counter-transference. Additionally, disclosure contributes to development of a trusting relationship between trainee and supervisor. This in turn enhances further disclosure. Verbal disclosure allows the trainee the opportunity to "think out loud" in the presence of another, with the trainee often recognizing links and meanings before receiving the supervisor's input. These accomplishments strengthen the trainee's growing sense of competence as a psychotherapist.

Certain conditions in the supervisory environment are prerequisites for self-disclosure. Winnicott (1965) developed the concept of the facilitating environment and the inseparability of the mother/infant dyad in relationship to development, while Kohut (1971) described the importance of selfobject experiences for the development and maintenance of the self. The supervisory situation ideally provides a facilitating environment for development of the trainee's clinical self, and the supervisor performs appropriate selfobject functions for learning. These sustaining features of the supervisory situation are essential conditions for self-disclosure. In more practical terms, the supervisor can lead the way by disclosing some of his or her own conflicts around the difficulties of a parallel clinical situation.

In describing the four domains of selfhood which emerge in infancy, Stern (1985) elucidates further the developmental context of disclosure and privacy. The third phase—development of the subjective sense of self—focuses on the sharing of subjective experience between self and other and the influencing of one another's subjective experience. Self-experiences are divided into three categories: the social self, the private self, and the disavowed self. The private self consists of experiences that have not been attuned with, shared, or reinforced, but that are not disavowed, and thus have access to language. Stern notes that there is enormous individual and cultural variability in what constitutes self-experience that is to be shared and that which is not, and that the boundary lines of the private domain shift and change with experience.

The trainee's domain of "private self" will be both individually and culturally determined and will likely change over the course of training. As the rhythm and flow of the supervisory interchange develops, the trainee's boundaries of privacy may become evident through the pattern of material that is routinely presented for discussion and that which is omitted. The supervisor's awareness of and sensitivity to the trainee's private self can facilitate a gradual shifting toward an optimal level of disclosure for learning, while avoiding intrusion and subsequent disavowal of portions of the trainee's self-experience as a psychotherapist.

What Trainees Do Not Disclose

A review of clinical material not disclosed in supervision, as reported by trainees with various levels of experience, reveals several common areas where conflicts about privacy and disclosure come to the fore. These situations are highlighted in this section and may serve as markers for predicting potential problem areas for trainees in supervision.

Countertransference

As we noted previously, discussion of the trainee's counterreactions to patients involves a high degree of self-disclosure and anxiety. Trainees feel embarrassed by intense sexual, angry, or hateful feelings that they experience toward patients. They view their feelings as unprofessional and inappropriate, rather than as valuable pieces of information that enhance understanding of both patient and therapist, as more experienced clinicians are likely to do. Trainees note particular difficulty in disclosing sexual feelings and may defend against the feelings or act out against them, with disastrous consequences for the therapy.

A second-year male resident reported the following experience: "I delayed sharing the degree of my sexual countertransference toward a very attractive and highly flirtatious young woman who appeared for therapy sessions wearing see-through shirts. I did not disclose my reactions, because I was afraid they were abnormal and unprofessional. The effects were catastrophic for the therapy. Although I eventually had the courage to share my feelings about this patient with my supervisor and he was very helpful and supportive, the full complexity of the transference and countertransference was not adequately explored, resulting in a technical error by me. I confronted the patient about a certain sexual disclosure she had made in therapy. Although my supervisor in retrospect agreed that my interpretation was very accurate, he felt that my intervention was premature. The patient terminated therapy in an angry manner. No one realized how uncomfortable and disturbed I was about this patient's behavior, probably because I did not adequately discuss my reactions in supervision."

A third-year female resident felt unable to disclose her erotic feelings toward a male patient: "I saw a very attractive man close to my age for 8 months in psychotherapy. Uncharacteristically, I slept in one morning and missed a session with the patient, which I did not recall until the angry patient called me later that day. I did not discuss my mistake with my supervisor, because I felt embarrassed by my irresponsibility. A few weeks later, to my chagrin, I repeated the same behavior of "forgetting" a session with the patient, who was by now livid. I then became aware of how sexually attracted I had been to this patient in recent months and had feared inadvertently revealing my feelings; thus the missed sessions. I felt too embarrassed to discuss the situation with my male supervisor, a difficulty that was compounded by a somewhat sexually charged atmosphere in recent supervisory sessions."

The reticence of trainees to discuss sexual issues with their supervisors raises implications for teaching. Supervisors may be advised to bring up general anxieties around erotic transference and countertransference (perhaps from their own experience) at some point in supervision without waiting for the trainee to initiate such a discussion. Increasing the trainee's awareness of intense feelings that can develop in the therapist during therapy can lead to fruitful discussion about ways to understand these reactions and thus to avoid acting on them. Given the recent public and professional attention that has been focused on patient-therapist sexual contact, such education can of course no longer be regarded as optional. Supervisors must also be sensitive to any sexualization of the trainee-supervisor relationship, which can severely inhibit disclosure and learning (Pope 1989).

Trainees who work with difficult patients in psychotherapy are likely to occasionally experience feelings of hate and anger (Groves 1978). A trainee may interpret these hating feelings as evidence that he or she is incompetent and unempathic, rather than as expectable reactions to the actual personality and behavior of the patient, based on an objective observation (Winnicott 1949). Beginning therapists may also have difficulty in sorting out the various complexities of projective identification that frequently occur with more primitive patients.

> A first-year resident found himself unable to discuss these common problems in supervision. He said, "My first psychotherapy patient was a woman with borderline personality disorder whom I began to see following her discharge from hospital. After the first month, she began to describe me as a "puppet," unable to be a real therapist because I was so unskilled and needed a supervisor. I felt out of my depth with the patient, and inside I silently agreed with her evaluation of me at times. I alternated between feeling depressed about my incompetence with her, and feeling hateful because she was free to verbally humiliate me while I had to remain calm and professional. I did not tell my supervisor about her comments, nor about my reactions, because I suspected that he would agree with her assessment of my skills."

Supervisors must be able to anticipate such possible counterreactions based on their knowledge of the dynamics of difficult patients, and to communicate to their trainees the acceptability and usefulness of examining personal feelings throughout the learning process.

Breaking Parameters of Therapy

Trainees bring with them certain expectations—sometimes in the form of rigid ideas—about how psychotherapy is supposed to proceed. For the novice therapist, these expectations may be derived from multiple sources, such as books, films, descriptions of therapy related by supervisors or other clinicians, or personal psychotherapy. The beginning therapist has little firsthand experience against which to measure the inevitable unexpected events that occur in psychotherapy. Trainees may assume that variations in behavior of either the patient or the therapist from their hypothesized "norms" represent failings on their part that must be kept secret. It is unfortunate that some of the most interesting and complex behaviors of patients and trainees may be omitted from discussion in supervision. In this way, rich material for learning about psychotherapy is lost. The following six examples illustrate interesting interactions that were not disclosed by trainees in supervision.

> In one session, I laughed *with* a patient at the ludicrousness of his suicide plan. I omitted this material from supervision as I was afraid that my supervisor would never understand the atmosphere in the session at that moment and would feel I was being very insensitive and unprofessional.

> A patient who had cried throughout her psychotherapy session hugged me as we stood up at the end of the appointment. Although disturbed, I was afraid to discuss the physical contact in supervision, because I was afraid I had done something to provoke it.

> I drifted off to sleep during a session with a wealthy patient who complained the entire session about her dog's problems. I was ashamed of my unprofessional behavior and did not discuss the

incident in supervision. However, the patient herself informed my supervisor, whom she had met previously, about my nap, although she refused to discuss the issue with me subsequently.

My psychotherapy patient kept me on the telephone for 30 minutes between sessions one week, but I reported to my supervisor that we had spoken only for a brief time, because I understood that it was important to keep contacts brief outside of sessions.

A patient who is an actor brought in a videotape of one of his performances that he wanted to discuss. I agreed to watch the video but omitted any mention of this incident in supervision because I wondered if I was doing "real" psychotherapy.

A new psychotherapy patient who had just moved to the area asked me if I could recommend a hairdresser, and I gave her an appropriate name. I was astounded when she appeared the following week with a haircut similar to mine. I was reluctant to tell my supervisor, because I suspected that I should not have responded to her request.

The trainee's perceptions of what constitutes clinical material lying outside the acceptable parameters of psychotherapy is to some degree individual. However, common themes among trainees are evident in their reluctance to disclose such interactions as out-of-session contacts, personal requests or questions from the patient, fees, gifts, hugs, compliments, and nonverbal communications from the patient such as diaries, paintings, or photographs. Supervisors can help trainees to explore some of their preconceptions about psychotherapy and emphasize the importance of understanding all types of interaction (including unexpected or embarrassing events) between patient and therapist. Supervisors can also model disclosure by revealing some of their own experiences of novel, amusing, embarrassing, or anxiety-provoking events from their practice as psychotherapists. More importantly, supervisors would do well to maintain a certain humility around the impact of some of these breaks in the "therapeutic frame." Most supervisors, if they look deeply into themselves, can recall instances where the unusual event had a surprising benevolent impact on the clinical hour. It is clear that the data are not complete on these matters of technique, within certain limits of safety and respect for the patients.

Theoretical "Correctness"

Many trainees identify with particular theoretical models during training and attempt to behave with patients in stereotyped ways that adhere to these models. For the inexperienced clinician, the result may resemble a caricature of, for example, the "blank screen" classical analyst or the warmly empathic self psychologist. Trainees may omit from discussion in supervision material or behavior that deviates from their current theoretical stance. In addition, trainees are often aware of their supervisor's theoretical biases and may modify material for presentation so as to avoid conflict with their supervisor's views. The following two examples illustrate trainee concerns with theoretical "correctness."

> I did not reveal to my supervisor my concerns about an incident when I was directive with a patient. The patient described having symptoms from a lump in his neck. I was concerned and suggested to the patient that he have it checked out. While I felt that my intervention was good for the patient, I felt some guilt that I was not being neutral and nondirective in the classic analytic style.

> I have a patient who attends experiential workshops that, at times, involve books and drawings that he brings in to discuss with me. I have never talked about this with my supervisor as I am afraid he will think I'm not doing "pure" dynamic psychotherapy. My supervisor tends to view such self-help activities outside of therapy as resistance, in contrast with my view that they are sometimes helpful adjuncts.

It is helpful for the supervisor to ask the trainee about his or her exposure to various theoretical models, including the theoretical orientation of previous supervisors, so that the current supervisor can form a picture of the trainee's attitudes and beliefs that influence behavior with patients. The supervisor's assistance in helping the trainee to view the patient from several theoretical perspectives, and avoidance of dogmatism, broadens the scope of material that is "safe" for the trainee to disclose. Trainees may feel caught between biological and psychological treatment modalities at times. This is illustrated in the following example, in which the trainee felt reluctant to disclose the use of concurrent medication with a psychotherapy patient.

> I have a patient with a personality disorder and intermittent symptoms of anxiety in ongoing psychotherapy. The patient began using small doses of benzodiazepines on a regular basis for years before starting therapy, and I have felt reluctant to stop the medication up until this point in time. I have never discussed his use of medication with my supervisor, mainly because I feel somewhat guilty using benzodiazepines in a palliative way, as if I'm tiding things over. I wonder if my keeping this "secret" is actually reinforcing the patient's sense of shame about needing medication, and perhaps limiting our consideration of other alternatives.

Conclusion

Supervision of psychotherapy remains a much understudied process, of vital importance to the profession. Perhaps one of the reasons for this has to do with the reluctance of supervisors and trainees to breach together the barriers to the highly personal and intimate process of psychotherapy, on the one hand, while needing to do just that to ensure the appropriate training of the clinician and the well-being of the patient in his or her care. In this chapter, we have explored some of the tensions around privacy and secrecy in supervision and have differentiated between healthy privacy and maladaptive secrecy in the supervisory situation.

Although most faculty members and students know that such secrecy and privacy exists, few ever address the issue beyond a knowing wink at supervisory meetings or at residency committees. We believe that there is value in sensitizing all parties to the interaction. In so doing, both supervisor and trainee can be increasingly confident about the developing competence of the neophyte clinician. With increasing trust, there is no need for the student to plunge into more pernicious secrecy out of fear of an unduly strict and moral set of rules that do not take into account the student's shame and impotence in the face of a clinical crunch. Because the patients who most invite the trainee to err, and to conceal those errors, are those patients who are dominated by shame and a sadistic superego, there is a risk that the parallel process will encourage similar harsh judgments in both therapist and supervisor around the work with these patients. When this happens, the stage is set for a disastrous outcome for the patient and for an unfortunate compromise in the clinical development of the trainee.

The same theories that inform the work with our patients around the development of healthy and pathological narcissism, autonomy and identity formation, and integrity of the self are brought to bear in the supervisory relationship. These theories can help supervisors and their students to acknowledge the value as well as the pitfalls that exist along the privacy/disclosure continuum in psychotherapy supervision.

References

Alonso A: The Quiet Profession: Supervisors of Psychotherapy. New York, Macmillan, 1985

Alonso A, Rutan JS: Shame and guilt in psychotherapy supervision. Psychotherapy 24:576–581, 1988a

Alonso A, Rutan JS: The experience of shame and restoration of self-respect in group therapy. Int J Group Psychotherapy 38:3–27, 1988b

Betcher RW, Zinberg NE: Supervision and privacy in psychotherapy training. Am J Psychiatry 147:796–803, 1988

Blatt S: Levels of object representation in anaclitic and introjective depression. Psychoanal Study Child 29:107–157, 1974

Brightman BK: Narcissistic issues in the training experience of the psychotherapist. International Journal of Psychoanalytic Psychotherapy 10:293–317, 1984–1985

Bromberg PM: The third ear, in Clinical Perspectives on the Supervision of Psychoanalysis and Psychotherapy. Edited by Caligor L, Bromberg PM, Meltzer JD. New York, Plenum, 1984

Chrzanowski G: Can psychoanalysis be taught?, in Clinical Perspectives on the Supervision of Psychoanalysis and Psychotherapy. Edited by Caligor L, Bromberg PM, Meltzer JD. New York, Plenum, 1984

Ford ESC: Being and becoming a psychotherapist: the search for identity. Am J Psychother 17:472–482, 1963

Freud S: On beginning the treatment (1913), in The Standard Edition of the Complete Psychological Works of Sigmund Freud, Vol 12. Edited by Strachey J. London, Hogarth Press, 1958, pp 135–156

Greenberg L: Supervision from the perspective of the supervisee, in Psychotherapy Supervision: Theory, Research, and Practice. Edited by Hess AK. New York, Wiley, 1980

Groves JE: Taking care of the hateful patient. N Engl J Med 298:883–887, 1978

Issacharoff A: Countertransference in supervision: therapeutic consequences for the supervisee, in Clinical Perspectives on the Supervision of Psychoanalysis and Psychotherapy. Edited by Caligor L, Bromberg PM, Meltzer JD. New York, Plenum, 1984

Josephs L: Self-disclosure in psychotherapy and the psychology of the self, in Self-Disclosure in the Therapeutic Relationship. Edited by Stricker G, Fisher M. New York, Plenum, 1990

Kohut H: The Analysis of the Self. New York, International Universities Press, 1971

Mahler MS, Pine F, Bergman A: The Psychological Birth of the Human Infant. New York, Basic Books, 1975

Morrison A: Shame, the ideal self, and narcissism. Contemporary Psychoanalysis 19:295–318, 1986

Pope KS: Teacher-student sexual intimacy, in Sexual Exploitation in Professional Relationships. Edited by Gabbard GO. Washington, DC, American Psychiatric Press, 1989, pp 163–176

Rustin M: The social organization of secrets: towards a sociology of psychoanalysis. International Review of Psychoanalysis 12:143–159, 1985

Stern DN: The Interpersonal World of the Infant. New York, Basic Books, 1985

VanBuskirk D: Identity development in the beginning psychiatrist, in Teaching Psychotherapy of Psychotic Patients. Edited by Semrad EV, VanBuskirk D. New York, Grune & Stratton, 1969

Winnicott DW: Hate in the countertransference. Int J Psychoanal 30:69–74, 1949

Winnicott DW: The Maturational Process and the Facilitating Environment. New York, International Universities Press, 1965

Zinberg NE: The private versus the public psychiatric interview. Am J Psychiatry 142:889–894, 1985

Chapter 14

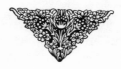

When Supervision May Fail: Difficulties and Impasses

Ronald Ruskin, M.D., F.R.C.P.C.

Education is not a college course, not a medical course, but a life course, for which the work of a few years under teachers is but a preparation. Whether you will be faithful to the end depends on the training before the start.

William Osler (1905/1945), "The Student Life," p. 400

Introduction: The Notion of Supervisory Infallibility

In "Analysis Terminable and Interminable," Freud (1937/1973) underlined the demanding role of the analyst who must possess "some kind of superiority, so that in certain analytic situations he can act as a model for his patient and in others as a teacher" (p. 248). Yet, in this superior position, Freud went on to say, something paradoxical and humbling may occur—that is, the task becomes one of those "'impossible' professions in which one can be quite sure of unsatisfying results."[1]

---

[1] The type of therapy and supervision referred to in this chapter is based on a model of individual, psychodynamically oriented therapy and supervision.

Can supervision, like analysis, be seen as an impossible or interminable task? The answer, at first, would seem clearly to be no. Traditionally the supervisor is the senior person, the expert-teacher who possesses objective academic knowledge and invaluable clinical experience, and the supervisee is the junior "neophyte" who does not yet have either the extent of knowledge nor the experience of the supervisor.

Solnit (1970) has described supervision as

> a process in which two or more people participate in a joint effort to establish, maintain, and/or elevate a level of performance . . . the supervisor possesses skills, experience, and understanding in excess of those possessed by the other participant, the supervisee." (p. 360)

Lebovici (1970) has suggested that "the supervisor sees better and elaborates better because he sees beyond the immediate and the ordinary." (p. 385). More recently, Levenson (1984) has argued that "there is something oddly infallible about the experience of doing psychotherapy supervision . . . when I supervise, *all is clear to me!*" (p. 153).

The notion of infallibility with regard to the supervisor's view of the "chaotic emotional experiences of the treatment sessions" (Arlow 1963, p. 593) must be critically reviewed, given that the supervisory situation contains anxieties of supervisor, supervisee, and patient. An underlying assumption that probably serves a defensive purpose and may at times distort the supervisory process is that the supervisor is (or gives the illusion of being) *above* experiencing anxiety or failure, knows best, and is absolutely objective. "This belief probably encourages methods that hinder, rather than facilitate, the supervisee's development . . . the supervisor often feels pressured to make knowledgeable remarks and the supervisee needs to present material naively" (Lesser 1984, p. 144). Furthermore, the notion of infallibility may permit the supervisor to enact a series of idealizations that protect and distance him or her from the possibility of critical and/or creative interaction with the supervisee. If the supervisor comes to accept this idealized experience of him- or herself as other than a representational quality, crucial self-analytic questioning and self-supervision may be diminished.

Freud (1937/1973) wrote of a need for a critical and corrective influence referring to periodic reanalysis of the analyst: "Every analyst should periodically—at intervals of 5 years or so—submit himself to analysis once more, without feeling ashamed of taking this step" (p. 249). Might the same be true for the supervisor? Indeed, to maintain and enhance their critical capacities, some analysts and therapists continue as supervisees in their own supervision well after the completion of training (Frijling-Schroeder 1970), while others regularly involve themselves in peer group consultations.[2] The subject of self-supervision has not often been reported. Adler (1972) has described his own experience.

> As a first-year psychiatric resident I became aware of a reaction when I worked with some difficult patients and felt particularly lost and helpless. I would have the thought, "If only my supervisor were here; he'd tell me what to do." Since he didn't appear at that moment, I would try something I recalled him discussing and demonstrating with a patient. Sometimes it would work, to my relief and delight, but often it would not . . . as my training proceeded, the syndrome . . . continued . . . it got worse . . . but the essence of the syndrome was the same: My helplessness with a patient, the summoning of an image of the omnipotent teacher who would have no trouble doing what I could not. (p. 316)

Adler (1972) concluded that feelings of helplessness and hopelessness were a necessary part of the burden a therapist had to bear. Interestingly, at the very time he experienced such "failure," there were trainees who turned to him as an idealized rescuer. Langs (1980) has discussed self-supervision and a self-supervisory attitude as a much neglected subject and an interminable process. He suggests, as did Freud, that "countertransferences were never entirely resolved, that they are an element, however small, in every interven-

---

[2] Ethical and legal pressures have increasingly exposed psychotherapy supervision (and ultimately the supervisor) to external review (see Chapter 2).

tion, and that both self-analysis and self-supervision are the major correctives to our best, though never perfect efforts" (pp. 123–124).

Manifest "Failure" in Psychotherapy and Supervision

Experiences of "failure" are common in psychotherapy and supervision, although not always accessible to self-analysis or discussion with colleagues. In supervision, the question of agency (i.e., who makes the original mistake) may be clear, agreed upon by both participants, and satisfactorily worked through. Alternatively, such mistakes or errors may be unclear, not apprehended by either participant, and only later recognized in some derivative form. At one end of a spectrum are "minor failures"—problems in technique, theory, or empathic responsiveness, mistakes in selection and/or treatment of "suitable psychotherapy cases," difficulty in grasping the dynamic unconscious, countertransference issues, gender and/or cultural issues, premature terminations, and occasional miscommunications between therapist and patient or therapist and supervisor that can be apprehended and resolved within the supervisory relationship. In midspectrum are "moderate failures"—disjunctions mentioned previously that have not been resolved, or others such as malignant regressions in therapy, therapeutic and supervisory impasses, substantial learning blocks (dumb spots), and countertransference problems (blind spots).

Traditionally, the onus falls upon the supervisor in his or her training role to facilitate and effect a resolution of this difficulty. In return, the supervisor may call upon a consultant or group (i.e., a peer or supervisors' group) to review the impasse and "supervise" the supervision. The sooner such "moderate failures" are noted and supervisory collaboration effected, the more likely a successful resolution. At the far end of this spectrum lie failures of such affective distress and magnitude that resolution within the supervisory relationship is impossible. Destructive countertransference acting-out behavior, inappropriate transgression of personal and/or sexual boundaries, incompetence or negligent professional behavior of the psychotherapy supervisee or supervisor, and the suicide of the patient may rank as "major failures," in contrast with minor and moderate "failures" previously mentioned. External authorities (e.g., the training director or institute administrator) must be involved at this stage to initiate appropriate responses that may include not only therapeutic interventions but also academic, legal, and disciplinary action.

"Major failures" are in fact tragedies within an institution teaching psychotherapy. Such events exert extensive and profound effects outside the supervisory relationship on the working ego, affective state, and self-esteem of many professionals at all levels of training. However, it is beyond the scope of this chapter to define, list, or discuss the ramifications of such "failures" comprehensively. Indeed, my purpose is to focus selectively on the experience of "failure" within supervision and to cite some commonly observed phenomena that require greater discussion and elaboration.

The frequency and nature of inadequacies or "failures" in psychotherapy supervision are not precisely known. Alonso (1985) has referred to supervisory impasses as occurring "occasionally," but there appears to be little research in this area and a consequent need for gathering and analyzing such data. In a widely cited study of residents' supervision, Perez and colleagues (1984) found that 11.5% of 157 residents experienced individual long-term therapy psychotherapy supervision as inadequate in quantity and quality.

Pate and Wolff (1990), following the earlier study by Perez and colleagues (1984), demonstrated that positive supervisory rapport, supervisor's teaching ability, and supervisor's fund of knowledge were "most determinant of a satisfactory supervisory experience" (p. 122). Indeed, Perez and colleagues (1984) found that the most highly rated characteristic of the supervisor's profile was "his or her capacity for developing *good rapport* with trainees" (p. 661).

If there is an atmosphere of trust and a mutuality of shared learning goals, the supervisory situation can be the preferred common area in which to study difficult therapeutic work. Fleming and Benedek (1983) parallel Freud's concept of the therapeutic alliance with that of the *learning alliance*—the supervisory working relationship that includes the acceptance of mutually shared goals and the "confidence that the expectations of teacher and learner can be satisfied" (p. 53). However, the learning alliance is a necessary but not sufficient condition for a positive supervisory process. Fleming and Benedek (1983) distinguish a further condition, "the expression of emotional resonance and intuitive understanding in a relationship" or rapport. What is "good" rapport or "bad" rapport is determined by the balance between members of each system and is "easily disturbed by responses from one party that do not meet the expectations which motivate the other party at a given moment" (p. 53).

Rapport and Good Enough Supervision

The term "good enough" has been appropriated from Winnicott's work on the relationship between mother and infant. In "Ego Integration in Child Development," Winnicott (1962/1985) refers to the "good enough mother *being* able to meet the needs of her infant at the beginning, and to meet these needs so well" (p. 57; italics added). Winnicott is referring to the adaptive and responsive function of maternal care and its converse—that is, "all the degrees and varieties of maternal failure" (p. 58). In failing to meet the omnipotence of the infant and make some sense of it, the mother may promote a compliance on the part of the infant that would be part of a false self.

Winnicott writes of the "personal growth" of the individual and the psychoanalyst as being "good enough" in his or her work with the patient. Although the analyst is not involved in child care, the concept of involvement in personal growth is as true for psychoanalytic work as it is for supervisory work. A number of writers have referred to the notion of good enough supervisors or good enough supervision (Alonso 1985; Brightman 1983; Everett and Striker 1990; Greben 1992; Pate and Wolff 1990; Ruskin 1992). Basic to all definitions seems to be what Greben (1992) refers to as a type of mutuality or reciprocity that fits in or combines with the other and leads to a "mutual trust." Such a good enough supervisory relationship allows for disclosure, expression of difference, a more genuine discussion of supervisory experience and "failures," and the consequent facilitation of learning and professional growth. It would appear that a good enough supervisory relationship is a precondition for satisfactory supervision. The absence of a good enough supervisory relationship may predispose toward failure.

▼ Supervision Failure: A Parallelism

A first-year resident met with his supervisor a number of times to discuss the selection of a suitable first case. The supervisor left the choice up to the resident, explaining to himself that this would give him the freedom and openness to select several cases from a waiting list and do assessments on his own. Because his supervisee was a neophyte therapist, the supervisor reasoned their sessions could be used to review basic principles of psychotherapy and to discuss papers, and let him find his own pace.

After several supervisory sessions had elapsed, the supervisor found himself disappointed that his supervisee had not engaged a case in therapy. The supervisor also began to feel somewhat critical of the resident's capacities as well as his own supervisory skills and wondered how this would look to other staff and supervisors. Feelings of anxiety, embarrassment, and some guilt about his "supervisory failure" alerted the supervisor to consider what he could do to help himself and his supervisee. In response to the supervisor's probing concern, the resident admitted in a rather low-keyed manner how anxious he was about doing a good assessment and maintaining a therapy case.

The supervisor became aware of a disconcerting pattern: the resident would present a new case, both would discuss the psychodynamics and suitability, and both would express initial therapeutic optimism. Shortly afterward, the patient would drop out. Gradually, as the supervisory relationship developed and a more open exchange of views occurred, the supervisor was struck by his countertransference resistance toward direct coassessment of cases and the resident's compliant and relatively low-keyed and uncritical attitude toward the selection process. The supervisor reflected on a parallel process: he had been trained in an analytic institute where candidates were required to find their own suitable cases—and where he had similarly struggled for a considerable period of time, vacillating between feelings of enthusiasm and despair in finding and then losing suitable cases. Subsequently, more active supervisory coassessments and interventions were helpful in finding a suitable therapy case that was maintained in psychotherapy.

Although the supervisor discussed the assessment process during supervision, he indicated (at least initially) a lack of interest in directly coassessing the psychotherapy cases with the resident. As the supervisory relationship developed, the supervisor quietly reflected on his own emotional responses (e.g., anxiety, embarrassment, fear of failure) to the supervisee's difficulty (Searles 1955). There is evidence of a parallelism and countertransference resistance between the supervisor's theoretical attitude toward assessment and that of his earlier supervisory experience during his analytic training, as well as the resident's particular difficulty. The supervisor was able to make use of his affective experience of "failure," which on one level acted as a signal to some corrective critical questions and action. Was this supervisory relationship good enough?

Arguably, the initial phase of supervision was not good enough. The supervisor did not appreciate that the resident's manifestly low-keyed approach and compliant and uncritical "false self" attitude toward selection protected him from anxiety. However, over time both participants were able to develop a certain mutuality and respect for each other, which led to a more genuine style of relating, comprising a discussion of the assessment process and their respective concerns about it. As Everett and Striker (1990) have observed,

> [The] supervisee can be viewed as struggling to preserve a sense of self, and thus erecting a "false self" to ward off the impingements of the supervisor and, at the same time, to please the supervisor. The supervisee's presentation of a case will thus always be, to a greater or lesser degree, a false one, designed to protect his or her "true self," or core, from the intrusions of the supervisor. (p. 13)

Opinion is divided as to whether it is better to have the supervisee carry out the initial series of assessments on his or her own without the intrusion of the psychotherapy supervisor, or whether the presence of an experienced psychotherapy supervisor may be invaluable in facilitating a psychotherapy assessment over time, particularly for a neophyte therapist. In the example "Supervision Failure: A Parallelism," the supervisor's affective responses to the supervisee within supervision initiated critical and corrective actions to avert "failure." It is important in cases like this to differentiate between psychoanalytic supervision and psychodynamic supervision in a university teaching hospital. In the former, there may be a tradition of privacy, autonomy, and confidentiality in the assessment phase of a new case in supervision. In the latter, there is the responsibility of the supervisor to have some direct knowledge of the patient.

It should be pointed out that the resident in this case example was also struggling with an observed phenomenon in therapy that affects many psychotherapists regardless of experience—premature psychotherapy termination. This is a relatively frequent occurrence, ranging from 12.5% of analytic cases seen by experienced analysts over a 2-year period (Erle and Goldberg 1984) to more than 50% of borderline cases in analysis or psychotherapy over a 4-year period (Waldinger and Gunderson 1984). In a study of premature psychotherapy termination, Frayn (1992) found that 20% of patients dropped out within 9 months or less following assessment and acceptance. Of these, 50% dropped out within 1 month. These figures are of considerable relevance when dealing with neophyte therapists. Premature termination (PT) cannot easily be avoided. It is often experienced as a disappointment or "failure" in the therapist's attempt to maintain a crucial self-esteem regulation. PT evokes therapist anxiety in the face of challenged psychotherapeutic competence and efficacy. Realistic discussions of the factors associated with this phenomenon may serve to reduce the therapist's sense of "failure." Frayn (1992) has suggested that a careful assessment carried out by the supervisors of the study sample consistently rated patients as initially having higher impairment scores than their supervisees. Less experienced supervisee-therapists tended to view their patients in a more optimistic light. It follows that more experienced supervisor-therapists view the patients with less denial and a greater awareness of structural deficits and characterological features and can impart this knowledge in supervision.

This example illustrates that vicissitudes of "failure" cannot be completely avoided. They are inherent within the supervisory process and outside of it. When dealt with appropriately, such "failures" represent a significant step toward addressing anxieties of supervisee (and supervisor), thus permitting new learning to take place.

I define the supervisee-supervisor dyad as a complex dynamic relationship that articulates at many different levels (Ekstein and Wallerstein 1972): that of the patient, the supervisee, the supervisor, and the administrator of the hospital. At each level, difficulties and impasses may arise and find their way into the supervision. If the supervisory relationship is experienced as "good enough," both supervisor and supervisee have the opportunity to empathically explore difficulties and therapeutic impasses. Alternatively, painful affects such as anxiety, helplessness, depression, shame, and guilt (Alonso and Rutan 1988), with associated defenses of isolation, denial, omnipotence, magical thinking, and grandiosity, may prevent a supervisory alliance.

The theme of omnipotence and grandiosity as a defense against helplessness, vulnerability, or failure is pervasive in the practice and supervision of psychotherapy as well as the identity of the psychotherapist (Alonso and Rutan 1988; Brightman 1983; Jones 1951; Mishne 1983; Ornstein 1968; Sharaf and Levinson 1967). If this theme is not addressed appropriately and early on in psychiatric training, the therapist may protect him- or herself against such affects by emotional distancing with patients, or adoption of a characterological attitude of unwavering self-certainty. In supervision, a humane mutual realization of the limitations of self, teachers, patients, and of paradigms in theory may offer greater solace and involvement in the search for understanding and the development of a professional identity. On the other hand, a denial of the experience of limitations or failure and a wish to remediate all unknowing renders the individual more susceptible to failure.

▼ Inability to Communicate Helplessness

A resident appeared self-assured and able to attend to his clinical duties without much support from staff supervisors. He radiated a manifest attitude of certainty and decisiveness. Initially, his self-sufficiency and optimism about his work seemed to indicate a high level of knowledge and confidence. However, as time went on, his supervisors began to experience anxiety. His patients did not like him, because he did not understand their concerns. The resident appeared to have an answer for everything. He rarely relied on his supervisors' clinical experience and seemed self-sufficient and somewhat contemptuous of the feelings and concerns of others. He had fixed ideas about treatment, and his clinical reports showed a distressing lack of organization and understanding of his patients. He also demonstrated a considerable lack of knowledge in many areas of psychiatry and an inability to assess and discuss his inadequacies.

When these problems were pointed out by his supervisors, the resident would at times disagree. When he was asked to reconsider or change certain medications, he would challenge his staff person as if he possessed equal medical knowledge. He did not appear to realize how he was alienating the staff; his supervisors strove to confront him in as constructive a manner as possible. Despite these interventions, the resident denied his learning problems. His inappropriate self-sufficiency placed his supervisors in a state of constant concern lest he make a major error.

Supervisory interventions did not impress on the resident that he was at risk of terminating his training program. A reluctant general agreement amongst supervisors indicated that his manifest defensive omnipotence and omniscience demonstrated that no learning or facilitation of change could occur. The postgraduate director expressed his distress about his department's inability to assist the resident but was forced to terminate his connection with the program.

This clinical anecdote of supervisee failure illustrates the character of the individual who cannot express helplessness or difficulty. When such qualities are firmly denied and externalized, empathic relatedness and the supervisory process may be stalemated and fail. In this instance, the supervisor can explore new ways of learning, but the supervisee cannot. As I mentioned previously, because no satisfactory supervisory resolution can occur, the magnitude of "major failure" extends beyond the supervisory relationship and impinges on the morale and self-esteem of the training program as a whole when a trainee is terminated.

The capacity for the initial experience of failure (whether real, anticipated, or imagined) to mobilize transference/countertransference acting-out behavior within the supervisory dyad, yet heighten narcissistic defenses against communication, has not often been discussed or reported in the literature. Ekstein and Wallerstein (1972) at times referred to such failures as "emergency situations." They differentiated between the internal conflict around inadequacy and helplessness in the patient or therapist and the externalization of this conflict into the supervisory relationship, obligating the supervisor to act or intercede with great alacrity. "The psychotherapist, in identifying with the helplessness to this degree, brings his own helplessness to the supervisor and asks the supervisor to take over" (Ekstein and Wallerstein 1972, p. 207).

▼ Manifest Supervisee Fear of Failure

A young woman hospitalized on the psychiatric ward with features of borderline personality and schizophrenic disorder developed a positive transference toward her therapist, a first-year male resident. The supervisor saw the patient together with the resident and assessed her to be a suitable case, but reviewed the possible development of an erotic transference. Therapy sessions were scheduled once weekly, and the patient received small amounts of antipsychotic medication. As sessions progressed, ward staff expressed concern about the degree to which the patient grew attached to the resident. To the resident, there appeared to be a growing confusion as to whether hospital staff felt this patient would be suitable for long-term psychotherapy. He ruminated over whether his kindness and reliability would provoke erotic behavior on the part of the patient. The resident then asked his supervisor to decide whether or not he should continue with this difficult case.

Complicating the resident's therapy were various ward staff who viewed him as being a "tyro" and at risk to have the patient deteriorate in therapy. In contrast, the supervisor reflected to the resident that although he was inexperienced, he showed considerable professional commitment with this patient and seemed reasonably knowledgeable in her management. In this case (as compared with the earlier example), supervisor and supervisee were able to directly discuss his anxiety related to his helplessness and fear of being implicated to arouse an erotic or regressive transference with his patient.

The resident asked his supervisor if he might predict the course of the erotic or regressive transference (which then seemed largely restricted to the patient's attachment, fondness, attentiveness, and preference for him). The supervisor explained that he could not know this. He added that the patient did not sound as if she were making unreasonable demands on her therapist and that the therapeutic situation and its boundaries appeared, for the time, stable. However, the supervisor asked if he might have the resident's permission to speak to a senior ward psychiatrist who had seen him work with this patient. Second, the supervisor inquired if he was embarrassed about his erotic feelings toward the patient, reassuring him that these feelings were normal. The resident explained that he had said nothing sexual whatsoever, but he worried that by being available to his patient he would increase her need for him. A consultation between the psychotherapy supervisor and the ward psychiatrist revealed a consistent level of support for the resident's work.

Subsequently, both supervisor and supervisee agreed that they would continue with this case and evaluate their progress. The supervisor reflected as a parallelism that he initially felt helpless for not acting in an absolute way. He had a fantasy that he should know exactly what to say—yet he knew very little! The supervisor's anxiety about therapy getting out of control had almost made him take over this case. To do this early in the therapy without any definite indications would devalue the therapist who already had expressed and was struggling with his feelings of inadequacy.

This supervisory juncture was a critical moment in the therapist's development (Rubin 1989).

Success in supervision requires that supervisee and supervisor allow themselves, at times, to communicate and experience the sense of *helplessness* or *not knowing*. The capacity to not know, or negative capability, referred to by Keats (Fitzpatrick-Hanly 1986) is paradoxically one of the essential characteristics of psychotherapy, supervision, and learning. A person allows him- or herself to not know in order to listen carefully to the other, to learn from the other. Perhaps this is also one of the steps leading to vicarious introspection or empathy. If the experience of helplessness is intolerable, then this process of "knowing" fails. It should be emphasized most strongly that an episode of helplessness or "failure" does not refer necessarily to a discrete failure in reality, but more accurately to how failure is linked to the internal representational world, dynamic conflicts, structural issues, and fantasies. Such failures do not reside simply within the patient or the therapist, but are also located in the representations of the supervisor and/or administrator of the psychotherapy training program.

▼ A Supervisor Failure

A senior resident presented her work to a junior supervisor who listened attentively but silently. Throughout her presentation, the supervisor adopted an "analytic attitude." He was unclear of some issues in therapy but decided to wait for more supervisory sessions when, he assumed, the issues would be clarified. In subsequent sessions, he began to experience an atmosphere of uneasiness, and the resident became increasingly silent. There were long empty pauses. Weeks later, she mentioned to her supervisor that he seemed dissatisfied with her work. The supervisor listened very carefully and attempted to address her concerns, but the resident felt he was quiet and essentially unresponsive. She thought she might see another supervisor.

Although he felt hurt, the supervisor realized the resident's criticisms were valid. The supervisor told the resident he would present their problem in a supervisory group coordinated by a senior supervisor. This required the supervisor to confront affects of self-exposure and shame before his peers in a potentially failing supervision. Fortunately, the group offered many helpful comments to the supervisor, the most simple of which was his increased participation and responsiveness in supervision, as well as the recognition that the resident was effective in registering her concerns within supervision. The supervisor realized that he had a theoretical resistance against "gratifying" the resident by talking too much. The supervisory group, led by a senior supervisor, offered the opportunity to the supervisor dyad to work through this temporary impasse. As a result of this encounter, both supervisor and supervisee felt less apprehensive, and supervision was able to continue and the impasse was largely resolved.

The use of a regular seminar (monthly or biweekly) to train new supervisors and serve as a forum for the work of more experienced supervisors has been generally accepted in many training institutions. Such training can help alleviate the difficulties or "failures" of new supervisors, who may find themselves closer to using a model that resembles therapy rather than supervision. Alonso (1985) suggests that such a supervisors' group develop a focus in research and theory on the supervisory process and refrain from dwelling exclusively on the problematic student, which may lead to avoidance of supervisory disclosure. Levy (1985) has advocated the use of a peer group of advanced psychiatric residents who discuss a taped psychotherapy session where the therapist shares recalled experiences with the group. Levy concluded, "peer group interactions . . . fostered their capacity to comprehend the multiple perspectives of the therapeutic interactions [and] . . . brought to light sound, new, and creative perspectives" (p. 511).

▼ A Treatment "Failure"

A bright first-year resident chose to work psychotherapeutically with difficult, regressed patients on an inpatient unit. However, despite his considerable therapeutic zeal, one patient failed to improve dramatically and was rehospitalized. It was clear to the supervisor that the patient and the resident shared excessive expectations of therapeutic change. The supervisor engaged in a gentle but open discussion of his wishes to "cure" the patient. At the same time, the supervisor disclosed his past experience in working with regressed hospital patients where he found himself accepting realistic but modest therapeutic gains.

Many years later, that resident recalled his supervision of a "treatment failure" as a pivotal point in his psychiatric training and a step toward a humane understanding of his grandiose professional aspirations as well as his own limitations.

Levels of Parallelism and the Experience of Failure

Numerous authors have described the existence of a parallel process between the therapist and patient, which refers to the capacity of the therapist to "play out" experiences or feelings which have been repressed in the patient and which the therapist relives in (and out of) supervision without awareness. Freud (1914/1973) originally wrote that "the patient *remembers* nothing of what is forgotten and repressed, but that he expresses it in *action*. He reproduces it not in his memory but in his behavior; he repeats it, without of course knowing that he is repeating it" (p. 150). Arlow (1963) has pointed out that while the patient oscillates between experiencing and reporting in sessions, the therapist oscillates between unconsciously identifying with the patient and observing him. Sachs and Shapiro (1976) referred to a crucial aspect of the therapist not only reporting what happens in sessions but also "demonstrating" what has happened. However, Sachs and Shapiro (1976) may err on the side of incompleteness when they suggest that this "often occurs when the novice therapist feels vulnerable and subject to anxiety" (p. 407).

Doehrman (1976) described in her instructive study that the parallel process works in more than one direction. Gediman and Wolkenfeld (1980) and Usher (1993) have observed that both supervisor and supervisee have a shared narcissistic vulnerability and that parallelism occurs in a complex multidirectional fashion. "Unresolved sectors of the analysts's and the supervisor's personalities . . . produce distortions and their sequelae in technique are . . . implicated in all parallel reenactments to one degree or another" (Gediman and Wolkenfeld 1980, p. 240). These experiences and enactments can originate from the most senior or influential individual within a training program. Such individuals, the "heads" from whom a certain measure of group allegiance and idealization is fostered, are also made more vulnerable at times by the considerable demands to maintain an apparent state of helpful superiority to their staff and patients. To an extent, they represent an external ego ideal (Freud 1921/1973) or how the self wishes he or she could be (Rycroft 1977). On another level, the administrative head represents an external conscience, capable of critical evaluation and approbation of trainees and supervisors. How does the attitude of the senior administrator reflect his or her own investment in psychotherapy training? How does the senior administrator deal with failure or helplessness?

▼ A Senior Administrative Failure

An administrative director, acknowledged as an expert in the long-term treatment of difficult schizophrenic patients, revealed to staff and residents that one of her well-known patients had recently committed suicide. In a grand rounds, the director explored the steps she had taken over many years to treat her patient and the events leading up to her suicide. The director fondly expressed the basic liking, mutual respect, and sense of fit that she and her patient maintained during the course of their long-term relationship. On many occasions, this physician had responded to her patient's depressive and suicidal crises and lived through her stages of helplessness, rage, and despair. She communicated her experience of her patient, existing in a state of unrelieved despair where suicide remained a distinct alternative. She also discussed how her patient had benefited from their therapeutic relationship, during which time the patient reached her highest level of functioning. Despite the relative success of their work together, this doctor exposed her inevitable feelings of loss and helplessness after the patient's completed suicide. Poignantly, she relayed the patient's fantasy of suicide bringing an end to the suffering she had chronically experienced since childhood.

This physician presented her case in a grand rounds open to all psychiatric hospital staff. The head of the outpatient service and the head of the Crisis Clinic, both senior analysts, acted as consultants who questioned and reviewed her findings. In light of her detailed presentation, neither clinician could offer a compelling therapeutic intervention that would have been, in retrospect, *more* efficacious than her own. At this point, the physician actively solicited staff comments about the management of this case. Several staff disclosed brief anecdotes of psychotherapy patients with abject and unmitigated psychic suffering. One staff person affirmed the inevitability of suicide in a therapeutic career and the importance of reviewing the therapist's feelings after the event (with a colleague, consultant, or supervisor), and then reported a recent patient suicide where he made himself available to the family during the process of mourning and attended the funeral. Such cases were not discussed with great finesse or elegant theoretical positions, but with the essential perplexing questions: "What had not been done? What more could have been done?" Although there was a muted expression of optimism in some cases, there was also the painful recognition that a small group of patients exists with whom continued therapeutic involvement is associated with suicidal behavior.

Does the administrator's exposure of her clinical work to two senior psychotherapy consultants in a grand rounds have any relevance to the supervisory process? It could be argued that this has nothing to do with supervision. On the other hand, both consultants were in a sense conducting an "open supervision" of the senior administrator's work before an audience of colleagues and students. Often the formats of grand rounds, continuing case seminars, and clinical presentations have within them elements of the supervisory process, namely a record of 1) the disclosure of the patient's behavior and experience in therapy, 2) the disclosure of the therapist's behavior and experience in therapy, and 3) the facilitation of an interactive experience of learning between the therapist-presenter and the supervisor-audience. Arlow (1963) has pointed out that the supervisory situation "may be compared to a kind of working through experience in which neurotic reactions to the role of therapist and to the process of empathy may be observed and studied phenomenologically" (p. 591). Arlow adds that the therapist "reexperiences in controlled and mitigated form the emotional impact which his patient has had upon him . . . and relives these emotional experiences in a circumscribed setting with his supervisor, who acts in the role of assistant, teacher, and *audience* " (p. 593).

Because these processes are ubiquitous, they are available for study, whether the format is that of the private supervisor/supervisee relationship behind closed doors or the open public presentation. Of course, it could well be argued that conditions of privacy and relative confidentiality favor greater disclosure, whether they are those of therapy or supervision.[3] Referring to the therapeutic interview, Zinberg (1987) points out that "the most compelling reason to breach . . . privacy . . . is to open up the process of research, evaluation, and teaching" (p. 1527).

In the case of "A Senior Administrative Failure," compelling reasons could be listed for the public presentation and supervisory process. First, there had been the recognition of a "major failure" in the completed suicide of a special patient treated by the senior administrator, which impinged on staff in the inpatient, outpatient, and emergency services who worked with this patient. Second, the senior administrator exposed her "failure" and turned to her audience for supervision. She expressed her helplessness for others to see and discuss with a sense of "basic safety" (Adler 1985). In a parallel fashion, the rounds stimulated personal disclosure and the reexperiencing of various affects of anxiety/helplessness in the context of therapists' professional self-esteem and competence. Third, this event facilitated a learning supervisory process based on an identification with a "head" who did not defend against vulnerability by omnipotent denial. Fourth, by exposing her work to the scrutiny of her colleagues and students, the administrator had enabled them to see that she could survive the hated destructive elements in her patient's suicide that had not destroyed her own internal good objects. She could continue to be a "good enough" therapist. Fifth, this public disclosure argued for the realistic anticipation and necessary preparation for failures in the lives of therapists and the capacity to develop resources for consultation and supervision for all involved.

---

[3] Granted, the supervisory aspect of this presentation can be criticized on other grounds (i.e., a lack of continuity—the administrator only presented this material during one session). Also, the audience in grand rounds could not conduct a complete examination of the patient's complex transference to her doctor over many years, or the doctor's equally complex countertransference to her patient. I believe that essential supervision can occur under the guise of rounds.

Latent Aspects of Failure in Supervision

The previous illustrations have been characterized by a reasonably clear or manifest recognition of difficulty or failure in supervision. One participant in the supervisory relationship has been able to identify a source of difficulty—an impasse, a failing—and draw attention to this problem within the supervision. However, it is possible that both participants are unable to experience, locate, or express this difficulty, and the difficulty persists. One example of this in supervision is the impasse that is "smooth" or "silent."

▼ A "Smooth Impasse"

An articulate, witty, and admiring third-year resident had a colorful manner of presentation. She seemed to have a fair grasp of the dynamics of her psychotherapy case and had the tendency to relate sessions in a comical fashion so that both she and her supervisor would often laugh. At times, the supervisor became uncomfortable with her admiration, the ease with which she presented and joked about her work, and her overfamiliarity with him. She asked about her supervisor's personal life and chatted animatedly about her own. Occasionally the supervisor felt himself irritated and manipulated by her comments. The supervisor wished to be seen as positively responsive, yet he did not want to enact a role of mutual disclosure. He refrained from answering many of her questions; in return, he did not ask her personal questions.

Somewhat concerned, the supervisor checked her progress with other psychotherapy supervisors and found her work was rated quite highly. The resident admitted she felt vulnerable with physically ill patients; she disclosed that a parent had been physically ill for a time. The supervisor had a similar history of a physically ill parent. In addition, the resident's psychotherapy patient had severe physical illness. The supervisor tried to understand the resident's comical presentations, which served to defend against her anxiety, and gently approached her countertransference experiences of anxiety with her patient.

Because the supervisor had somewhat similar countertransference anxieties and characterological responses (i.e., joking), this and other issues were not fully engaged in supervision. On a manifest level, supervision was felt to be positive and enjoyable, if not a pleasant relief from the humdrum and sturm und drang of clinical work. After a year of supervision, the resident continued to speak admiringly of her supervisor. Her supervisor continued to experience the supervision as a reassuring and pleasant confirmation of the smoothness of their fit that made him at times vaguely uneasy.

The supervisory relationship with the resident seemed to move along some dimensions very well: she was able to maintain a difficult physically ill patient in psychotherapy and discuss the course of therapy and her interventions. She was highly rated as a psychotherapy trainee. In retrospect, however, the supervisor felt as if he were missing something in not being more questioning, particularly with the resident's flattering admiration of him. After their supervision terminated, they both gave each other good evaluations. The supervisor reflected more carefully on how difficult it had seemed for either of them to challenge one other and risk losing the other's needed reassurance, approval, and mirroring responsiveness.

"Smooth" or "silent" impasses may occur more often than both participants in the supervisory relationship care to realize. Because of the need to establish an agreeable "false self" relationship, certain portions of supervisory work may be disavowed or denied. In a similar fashion, certain paradigms of psychotherapy, the limits of knowledge, and the capacity to know freely may remain unencountered within the supervisory relationship, and an important aspect of supervision may fail.

Paradigms of Psychotherapy Based on "Failure"

The supervisor is in a preferred and intimate position with the supervisee to review the human capacity to repetitively "fail" the other. The paradigm of "failure" is inherent in all relationships and begins at birth. Stern (1985) states that the infant is readily available to socially interact with the primary caregiver. From birth to 2–3 months during the emergent sense of self, research indicates that aspects of people and/or things can be experienced directly as categorical affects (e.g., anger, sadness, happiness) and others as vitality affects that may be construed as soothing or relaxing (Stern 1985). If the caregiver cannot offer vitality affects, "failure" may occur. Broucek (1991) has suggested that "efficacy of the infant's efforts vis-à-vis the world . . . depends on sensitive and 'good enough' maternal responsiveness. To the extent that the mother-child interaction fails to support and sustain a sense of efficacy, the primitive sense of self may be failed or 'damaged'" (p. 28).

Object relations theorists write about patients in whom therapeutic regression occurs and where there is a sense of continued helplessness for periods of time. The patient may often state that there is "some fault or defect in them" or something has irretrievably "gone wrong" (Balint 1968, p. 89). During these states of helplessness or "apparent failure," the analyst is cautioned to "avoid becoming or even appearing in the eyes of his patient the opposite, that is, 'omnipotent.'" (p. 89). As Winnicott (1963/1985) put it,

> In innumerable ways we meet our patients' needs because we know what the patient is feeling like, more or less, and we can find the equivalent of the patient in ourselves. What we have in ourselves we can project, and find in the patient. All this is done *silently,* and the patient usually remains unaware of what we do well, but becomes aware of the part we play when things go wrong. It is when we *fail* in these respects that the patient reacts to the unpredictable and suffers a break in the continuity of his going on being. (p. 250)

Winnicott goes on to say, "In the end the patient uses the analyst's failures, often quite small ones . . . so in the end we succeed by failing . . . " (p. 258).

Kohut (1984) extensively uses the concept of "failure" in his work on narcissism. He writes that "the analytic process will focus on . . . the recognition of the *failures* of the child's oedipal selfobjects" (p. 5). By this, Kohut refers to the inevitable appearance of certain narcissistic or selfobject transferences in which the patient reexperiences "failures" within the psychoanalytic work that can lead to a successful restoration.

Freud was perhaps the first to point out the recurrent nature of the fear of failure as a potent organizer of psychic life. Certain anxiety dreams (for example, Freud 1900/1973) illustrate this clearly:

> Everyone who has passed the matriculation examination at the end of his school studies complains of the obstinacy with which he is pursued by anxiety-dreams of having failed, or of being obliged to take the examination again, etc. In the case of those who have obtained a University degree, this typical dream is replaced by another one which represents them as having failed in their University Finals; and it is in vain that they object, even while they are still asleep, that for years they have been practising medicine or working as University lecturers or heads of offices. (pp. 273–274)

The dynamic context of failure in a supervisee's patient is central to understanding underlying conflict and, to a degree, can be reassuringly objectified within supervision. Failure as a paradigm is a necessary construct in psychotherapeutic work and supervision, because it reflects a phenomenon that, regardless of theoretical orientation, alerts the other to a crucial organizing structure and series of affects.

However, full disclosure and discussion may be prevented since supervision is experienced as critical evaluation (DeBell 1963). Supervisee fears of failure along with substantial learning regressions may be evident. Anxiety dreams are not unusual in a supervisee's experience (see Chapter 7), although it may be a more common experience for psychotherapy trainees and analytic candidates to discuss their disappointments with classmates rather than supervisors.

▼ Regression of the Student

A postgraduate student was a candidate in a psychotherapy program and had not as yet found her first control case. She had made contact with several patients who could not pay a reduced fee. When she presented assessments of her cases to her supervisor, whom she knew to be a kind and accepting individual, she nevertheless was struck by a cruel glint in his eyes when he listened carefully as if he were laughing secretly at her and thinking to himself how stupid she was. She felt too embarrassed to bring this up to him but told her classmates, who reassured her until she found her first case.

The student's failure to find a suitable case mobilized anxiety and led to a brief regressive experience of her supervisor as persecutor. Her classmates and friends were chosen to stabilize her precarious self-esteem.

Limits of Knowledge: Failure of Theory/Theory of Failure

A further area of "failure" occurs when a given psychological theory fails to offer sufficient explanation or prediction with a given patient. Polanyi (1958) wrote, "a theory . . . is objective knowledge in so far as it is *not I,* but the theory, which is proved right or wrong when I use such knowledge" (p. 4). As therapist-teachers, we invest in theories of behavior and seek confirmation in our concepts of what will lead to successful outcome. As Kuhn (1962) stated, experiences of "failure" are "anomalies or violations of expectation . . . *and . . .* need detailed study, as does the emergence of the crises that may be induced by repeated failure to make an anomaly conform" (p. xi).[4] The supervisor is in the position to facilitate an inclusive position and convey a tolerance for multiple theories by saying, "Each theory adds something new to our theoretical understanding" (Pine 1988, p. 571).[5] Alternatively, he or she may approach an exclusive position

----

[4] "Normal science . . . often suppresses fundamental novelties because they are necessarily subversive of its basic commitments . . . a normal problem, one that ought to be solvable by known rules and procedures, resists the reiterated onslaught of the ablest members of the group within whose competence it falls." (Kuhn 1962, p. 5)

[5] "As scientists, psychoanalytic clinicians work under a self-expectation to be true to the phenomena, to be servants to the data, to be reporters of the

that favors developing competence and expertise in one theory at the expense of another. Both inclusive and exclusive approaches have certain advantages and disadvantages. The use of multiple theories may offer too much initial confusion to the supervisee or suggest a superficial type of imitative learning (Fleming and Benedek 1983; Ornstein 1968) or "theoretical dilettantism." On the other hand, the supervisor's rigorous approval of one theory may not be applicable to a specific patient and may discourage the supervisee from working with another theory that he or she wants to increasingly understand and implement.

In the preface to their monograph on supervision, Ekstein and Wallerstein (1972) acknowledged that "we no longer operate within so comfortably shared a set of common psychological assumptions about how the mind hangs together" (p. xvi). More than two decades later, competition in the therapeutic marketplace is arguably more vigorous along with a challenge to therapeutic efficacy. As Gabbard (1990) describes it, a "more sensible solution is to become familiar with the phenomena described by all major theories and to focus on each perspective as it is clinically appropriate with a given patient." (p. 42). What happens if the supervisor is not conversant with or rejects other theoretical approaches? Does this not have an effect on the success or failure of professional identification and learning of the psychotherapy supervisee? How does the psychotherapy supervisor contend with the division of biological and psychodynamic approaches within the supervisee's own patient?

Gabbard (1992) explains that "much of the polarization between biological and psychodynamic perspectives arises from a *failure* to appreciate the complex relationships between psychosocial and neurophysiological factors in the etiology and the pathogenesis of psychiatric disorders" (p. 991). These questions of theory selection within psychodynamic psychotherapy and the approach to integra-

---

observed. This presses in the direction of openmindedness. But as professionals, psychoanalytic clinicians work under a self-expectation to be knowledgeable, to be expert in a body of knowledge they can apply in the relief of psychic distress. Patients come to us, and pay us, to be experts, not scientists. This presses in the direction of closure." (Pine 1988, p. 577)

tion of biological and psychodynamic perspectives—not either/or but and/also—may be meaningfully addressed within the supervisory relationship. Stein (1991) has suggested that the theory used by the psychoanalyst or psychodynamic therapist may "influence the analyst's countertransference and affect clinical judgment" (p. 333).

▼ **Two Supervisors and a Patient**

A patient with a difficult characterological disorder who had been abandoned as a young child was seen in psychotherapy by a supervisee who saw a supervisor, a classical analyst. After several differences of opinion, the patient became enraged, suicidal, and noncompliant in therapy with her therapist. The supervisee, because of a treatment impasse with her patient, referred the patient to consultation with a second consultant-supervisor who used a self psychological approach. In discussion with the classical analyst, the supervisee believed she should terminate her case. However, in discussions with the self psychological consultant, he suggested trying to continue therapy (albeit with an enraged and regressed patient) in an attempt to work on the impasse.

In this instance, the use of alternate theories permitted two well-qualified supervisors to differ radically in their treatment recommendations. One supervisory contact led to an abrupt termination, the other supervisory consultation to continued involvement.

The Capacity to Know Freely

One of the tasks of supervision is to encourage the supervisee to be able to develop the capacity to reflect on his or her work. In this sense, the supervisee is able to be supervised by the supervisor, but also to be supervised by him- or herself. In the presence of the supervisor, does the supervisee feel entitled to know and to experience and express his or her own thoughts? The preferred circumstance for this situation appears to be when the supervisory relationship is "good enough."

Symington (1990) has defined two types of knowing that have

relevance for the supervisory process. Intellectual knowing is defined as "knowing *about* someone or something"; affective or emotional knowing is "knowing someone or something directly." (p. 100; italics in original). The difference between intellectual knowledge and emotional knowledge is the difference between knowing a fact and knowing an experience. Although intellectual knowing may come with intelligence, observation, and reading, emotional knowledge is more difficult to come by. A person has to expose his or her true self, and this "is painful and therefore resisted" (Symington 1990, p. 100).

Psychotherapy supervision may fail if only intellectual knowledge is imparted to the supervisee. In this argument, supervisory experience has the opportunity to directly influence the supervisee through access to his or her emotional knowledge. It seems that the supervisory experience may be most profoundly realized and potentially liberating when both intellectual and emotional knowing occur.

Conclusion

Experiences of difficulty and failure are ubiquitous in psychotherapy. Empathic recognition of the dialogue of "failure" within supervision may offer the participants the potential to work on such problems without seriously lowering their self-esteem and competence. The supervisor is in an intimate and regulatory position in a psychotherapy teaching program. The supervisor/supervisee dyad functions as a complex dynamic relationship at many levels—that of the patient proper, the supervisee, the supervisor, and the administrator of the hospital. At each level, difficulties or impasses may arise and find their way into supervision. If the supervisory relationship is experienced as "good enough," there is the opportunity for both supervisor and supervisee to empathically explore difficulties and therapeutic impasses. Alternatively, painful affects such as helplessness, shame, and humiliation (with associated defenses) may prevent supervisory disclosure and lead to greater failure. I have reviewed some manifest aspects of supervisory "failure" that can be clearly recognized and contrasted them with more subtle or latent aspects of "failure" in supervision. The "good enough" supervisory relationship appears to be the preferred situation in which learning can occur.

References

Adler G: Borderline Psychopathology and Its Treatment. New York, Jason Aronson, 1985

Adler G: Helplessness in the helper. Br J Med Psychol 45:315–322, 1972

Alonso A: The Quiet Profession: Supervisors of Psychotherapy. New York, Macmillan, 1985

Alonso A, Rutan JS: Shame and guilt in psychotherapy supervision. Psychotherapy 25:576–581, 1988

Arlow JA: The supervisory situation. J Am Psychoanal Assoc 11:576–594, 1963

Balint M: The Basic Fault: Therapeutic Aspects of Regression. London, Brunner/Mazel, 1968

Brightman B: Narcissistic issues in the training experience of the psychotherapist. International Journal of Psychoanalytic Psychotherapy 12:112–121, 1983

Broucek FJ: Shame and the Self. New York, Guilford, 1991, pp 28–31

DeBell DE: A critical digest of the literature on psychoanalytic supervision. J Am Psychoanal Assoc 2:546–575, 1963

Doehrman M: Parallel processes in supervised psychotherapy. Bull Menninger Clin 40:3–104, 1976

Ekstein R, Wallerstein RS: The Teaching and Learning of Psychotherapy, 2nd Edition. New York, International Universities Press, 1972

Erle J, Goldberg D: Observations on assessment of analyzability by experienced analysts. Psychoanal Q 53(3):501–503, 1984

Everett PR, Striker G: Selection of patients for psychotherapy supervision, in Psychoanalytic Approaches to Supervision. Edited by Lane RC. New York, Brunner/Mazel, 1990, pp 9–24

Fitzpatrick-Hanly MA: Keats' oral imagination. Psychoanal Q 55:618–639, 1986

Fleming J, Benedek TF: Psychoanalytic Supervision: A Method of Clinical Teaching, 2nd Edition. New York, International Universities Press, 1983

Frayn DA: Assessment factors associated with premature psychotherapy termination. Am J Psychother 46(2):250–261, 1992

Freud S: The interpretation of dreams (1900), in The Standard Edition of the Complete Psychological Works of Sigmund Freud, Vol 4. Translated and edited by Strachey J. London, Hogarth Press, 1973, pp 273–274

Freud S: Remembering, repeating, and working-through (further recommendations on the technique of psychoanalysis II [1914]), in The Standard Edition of the Complete Psychological Works of Sigmund Freud, Vol 12. Translated and edited by Strachey J. London, Hogarth Press, 1973, pp 141–151

Freud S: Group psychology and the analysis of the ego (1921), in The Standard Edition of the Complete Psychological Works of Sigmund Freud, Vol 18. Translated and edited by Strachey J. London, Hogarth Press, 1973, pp 67–143

Freud S: Analysis terminable and interminable (1937), in The Standard Edition of the Complete Psychological Works of Sigmund Freud, Vol 23. Translated and edited by Strachey J. London, Hogarth Press, 1973, pp 216–253

Frijling-Schroeder: On individual supervision. Int J Psychoanal 51:363–370, 1970

Gabbard GO: Psychodynamic psychiatry in the "decade of the brain." Am J Psychiatry 149:991–998, 1992

Gabbard GO: Psychodynamic Psychiatry in Clinical Practice. Washington, DC, American Psychiatric Press, 1990

Gediman HK, Wolkenfeld F: The parallelism phenomenon in psychoanalysis and supervision: its reconsideration as a triadic system. Psychoanal Q 49:234–255, 1980

Greben SE: Significant aspects of the supervisor-supervisee relationship. Paper presented at the 42nd annual meeting of the Canadian Psychiatric Association, Montreal, Quebec, September 1992

Jones E: The God complex, in Essays in Applied Psychoanalysis, Vol 2. London, Hogarth Press, 1951, pp 244–265

Kohut H: in How Does Analysis Cure? Edited by Goldberg A with collaboration of Stepansky P. Chicago, IL, University of Chicago Press, 1984, pp 5–6

Kuhn TS: The Structure of Scientific Revolutions. Chicago, IL, University of Chicago Press, 1962

Langs R: Supervision and the bipersonal field, in Psychotherapy Supervision, Theory, Research, and Practice. Edited by Hess AK. New York, John Wiley, 1980, pp 103–125

Lebovici S: Technical remarks on the supervision of psychoanalytic treatment. Int J Psychoanal 51:385–392, 1970

Lesser R: Supervision: illusions, anxieties, and questions, in Clinical Perspectives on the Supervision of Psychoanalysis and Psychotherapy. Edited by Bromberg PM, Meltzer JD. New York, Plenum, 1984, pp 143–152

Levenson E: Follow the fox, in Clinical Perspectives on the Supervision of Psychoanalysis and Psychotherapy. Edited by Bromberg PM, Meltzer JD. New York, Plenum, 1984, pp 153–167

Levy J: Learning to comprehend the multiple perspectives of psychotherapeutic interventions. Can J Psychiatry 30:504–512, 1985

Mishne HL: Narcissistic vulnerability of the younger student: the need for non-confrontation empathic supervision. The Clinical Supervisor 1(2):3–12, 1983

Ornstein PH: Sorcerer's apprentice: the initial phase of training. Education in Psychiatry 9:293–315, 1968

Osler W: The student life (1905), in Aequanimitas, With Other Addresses to Medical Students, Nurses and Practitioners of Medicine, 3rd Edition. Philadelphia, PA, Blakiston, 1945, pp 397–423

Pate LA, Wolff TK: Supervision: the residents' perspective. Academic Psychiatry 14:122–138, 1990

Perez EL, Krul LE, Kapoor R: The teaching of psychotherapy in Canadian residency programs: residents' perceptions. Can J Psychiatry 29:658–664, 1984

Pine F: The four psychologies of psychoanalysis and their place in clinical work. J Am Psychoanal Assoc 36:571–596, 1988

Polanyi M: Personal Knowledge: Towards a Post-Critical Philosophy. Chicago, IL, University of Chicago Press, 1958

Rubin SS: At the border of supervision: critical moments in psychotherapists' development. Am J Psychother 43:387–397, 1989

Ruskin R: When supervision may fail: difficulties and impasses. Paper presented at the 42nd annual meeting of the Canadian Psychiatric Association, Montreal, Quebec, September 1992

Rycroft C: A Critical Dictionary of Psychoanalysis. Middlesex, England, Penguin, 1977

Sachs DM, Shapiro SH: On parallel process in therapy and teaching. Psychoanal Q 45:394–415, 1976

Searles HF: The informational value of the supervisor's emotional experience. Psychiatry 18:135–146, 1955

Sharaf MR, Levinson D: The quest for omnipotence in professional training. Int J Psychiatry 4:426–442, 1967

Solnit AJ: Learning from psychoanalytic supervision. Int J Psychoanal 51:359–362, 1970

Stein S: The influence of theory on the psychoanalyst's countertransference. Int J Psychoanal 72:325–334, 1991

Stern DN: The Interpersonal World of the Infant. New York, Basic Books, 1985

Symington N: The possibility of human freedom and its transmission (with particular reference to the thought of Bion). Int J Psychoanal 71:95–106, 1990

Usher SE: Introduction to Psychodynamic Psychotherapy Technique. Madison, CT, International Universities Press, 1993

Waldinger R, Gunderson J: Completed psychotherapies with borderline patients. Am J Psychother 38:190–202, 1984

Winnicott DW: Ego integration in child development (1962), in The Maturational Processes and the Facilitating Environment. London, Hogarth Press, 1985, pp 56–63

Winnicott DW: Dependence in infant-care, in child-care, and in the psychoanalytic setting (1963), in The Maturational Processes and the Facilitating Environment. London, Hogarth Press, 1985, pp 249–259

Zinberg NE: Elements of the private therapeutic interview. Am J Psychiatry 144:1527–1533, 1987

Index

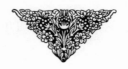

Page numbers printed in **boldface** type refer to tables or figures.

Acceptance, anxieties over, 66–67

Accuracy, importance of authenticity versus, in supervision, 214

Association of American Medical Colleges (AAMC) Faculty Roster data base, underrepresentation of cultural groups on, 65

Audiotapes
in development of psychotherapy supervisor, 196
ethical issues in use of, 20
in family therapy supervision, 124

Authenticity, importance of accuracy versus, in supervision, 214

Autonomy
in dealing with psychotic patients, 143
and identity formation, 219–220

Battered Women (self-help group), 23

Berlin Institute of Psychoanalysis, 190

Biopsychosocial model of treatment, 76

"Borrowed servant" doctrine, 26

Bowenian therapy, 122

Brief therapy model, 122

Canada, dimensions of cultural experience in, 63–64

Cheerleading strategies as form of validation, 172

Choice point analysis, 107–108

Closed-door model of supervision, 17–22

Cognitive-behavioral model, 165–186
clinical skills as goal of supervision in, 167–170, **169–170**
methods of supervision, strategies and procedures, 170

Cognitive-behavioral model
    (continued)
  models of supervision,
      179–181
    accepting dialectical
        philosophy,
        181–182
    accepting fallibility of
        therapists, 183–184
    agreeing to accept
        diversity, 185
    avoiding role of
        intermediary, 185
    helping each other
        understand and
        conceptualize patient
        behavior, 184–185
    observing personal limits
        when conducting
        therapy, 182–183
  skills training, 173
    response acquisition
        procedures, 174–175
    response disinhibition
        procedures, 176–178
    response inhibition
        procedures, 178–179
    response shaping and
        strengthening
        procedures,
        175–176
  supervisory problem solving,
      172–173
  validation in, 170–172
Cohen v. State of New York,
    24–25
Communication

  in development of
      psychotherapy
      supervision, 202
  impact of gender on, 41–43
  theory of, 123
Competence, anxieties over,
    66–67
Confidentiality. *See also* Privacy
  concerns of, in family
      therapy supervision, 123
  in dealing with psychotic
      patients, 143
  value of, in psychotherapy,
      17–18
Conflicts, externalizing causes
    of, 121
Cotherapy
  with dyadic supervision,
      110–111
  of psychotic patients, 143–144
Countertransference. *See also*
    Transference
  issues related to, 108–109
  mirroring of, with psychotic
      patients, 144–145
  in psychotherapy
      supervision, 222–225
Crisis psychotherapy
    supervision. *See*
    Emergency/crisis
    psychotherapy supervision
Cultural issues in
    psychotherapy supervision,
    53–55
  definition of culture in, 55
  dimensions of, in Canada
      and United States, 63–64

early studies of
    patient-therapist
    interaction, 56–58
impact of cultural
    differences, 60–61
professional
    underrepresentation of
    cultural groups, 64–65
psychotherapy training, 58–60
sense of self in, 61–62

Dialectical behavior therapy
    (DBT), 166
Dialectical philosophy,
    acceptance of, 181–182
Dialectical supervision
    framework, 180–181
Didactic learning, 99
Disclosure versus privacy in
    psychotherapy supervision,
    211–229
nondisclosures, 222–228
theoretical and
        developmental
        underpinnings, 217–222
Dual relationships, concern
    about, in ethical guidelines,
    31, 32–36
Dyadic supervision, 110–111

Electrically recorded interview,
    19
Emergency/crisis
    psychotherapy supervision,
    151–163
definition of emergency and
    crisis in, 151

fundamental characteristics
    of, 155
opportunities offered by
    countertransference issues,
    152–163
hostile and unempathic
    responses, 152–153
omnipotent control, 152,
    153–154
passivity, 152, 154
psychodynamic life
    narratives in, 155–157
Emotional knowledge, 257
Empathic listening in
    emergency/crisis
    intervention, 152–153,
    154–155
Ethical issues in psychotherapy
    supervision, 11–36. *See also*
    Legal aspects of supervision
dual relationships in, 31,
    32–36
and fiduciary obligation,
    31–36
identity crisis in, 22–24
literature on, 29–31
and standard of care, 27–29
video technology and
    closed-door model of
    supervision in, 17–22
Experiential group
    participation, 99

Failure
    fear of, 242–244
    latent aspects of, in
        supervision, 250–251

Failure *(continued)*
  paradigms of psychotherapy
    based on, 251–254
Family concerns of psychotic
  patients, 142–143
Family therapy, comparisons
  between individual
  psychotherapy and,
  127–128
Family therapy supervision,
  121–132
  areas of focus in, 129–130
  attitude of supervisee in,
    128–129
  audiotapes in, 124
  confidentiality concerns in,
    123
  importance of, 131–132
  isomorphism in, 128
  levels of training in, 122
  live, 124–126
  need for group of students
    in, 126–127
  need for support in, 131
  one-way mirror in,
    124–126
  opportunities offered by,
    130–131
  process notes in, 123–124
  role-playing in, 127
  simulation in, 127
  transference/counter-
    transference
    phenomena in, 128
  types of teaching in, 122
  videotapes in, 124
Federal Torts Claim Act, 25

Fiduciary obligation of
  psychotherapy supervisor,
  31–36
Foreign medical graduates,
  experiences of, 63–64
Free association, 16
Functional family therapy, 122

Gender issues in supervision
  consenting adults in, 46–47
  impact of gender on
    communication, 41–43
  need to identify with
    supervisor, 45–46
  recommendations in, 49–50
  in resident selection and
    evaluation of
    supervisors, 47–49
  and sexual abuse of patients,
    47
  sexual embarrassment in, 47
  supervisor-trainee
    boundaries in, 43–44
  supervisor-trainee
    competitiveness in,
    44–45
Group demoralization and
  disintegration, 102–103
Group instability, phenomenon
  of, 103
Group therapy supervision,
  99–117
  behavioral methods in, 174
  choice point analysis in,
    107–108
  isomorphy in, 105–106
  models of, 109–110

dyadic, 110–111
supervision group,
113–115
triadic, 112–113
observation, 115–116
task of, and supervisory
relationship, 103–109
trainee's reactions to unique
aspects of, 100–103

Helplessness, inability to
communicate, 240–242
Hospitalization of psychotic
patient, 145–146
Hostility as countertransference
issue, 152
Hungarian method of
psychotherapy supervision,
14–15, 16

Identity formation, and
autonomy, 219–220
Incompetence, and language,
68–69
Indirect techniques, 122
Individual psychotherapy,
comparisons between
family therapy, 127–128
Integrative psychodynamic, 122
Intellectual knowing, 257
Interracial analysis, 57–58
Intersubjectivity, and
development of self,
220–222
In vivo modeling in behavioral
methods, 174–175

Isomorphism in family therapy
supervision, 105–106, 123,
128

Knowledge
limits of, 254–256
types of, 256–257

Language
anxieties over competence
and acceptance, 66–67
difficulty in finding suitable
case, 67–68
incompetence, 68–69
linguistic competence and
anxiety, 65–66
Learning alliance, 235–236
establishment of, in group
psychotherapy
supervision, 104
Legal aspects of supervision,
11–14, 24–27. *See also*
Ethical issues in
psychotherapy supervision
and malpractice, 12–13, 23–24
Linear supervision, **93**
Live supervision in family
therapy supervision,
124–126

Malpractice litigation
economic incentives in, 23–24
against mental health
professionals, 12–13
Manifest failure in
psychotherapy and
supervision, 234–236

Marston v. Minneapolis Clinic of Psychiatry, 26
Medical school, clinical training in, 74
Medical teaching, person versus case in, 137–139
Medication dose, reduced, 147
Mental health professionals
  ethical principles for, 13
  malpractice claims against, 12–13
Mentoring programs, 33–34
Milan approach, 122
Mirroring transference and countertransference, 144–145
Modeling in behavioral methods, 174–175

Narcissism, 218

Object relations therapy, 121–122
  shame in, 218
Observation of group therapy, 99, 115–116
Omnipotent control as countertransference issue, 152, 153–154
One-way mirror
  ethics in use of, 20
  in family therapy supervision, 124–126
Overinvolvement, 161–162

Parallelism, levels of, and experience of failure, 246–249
Parallel process, 123
Passivity as countertransference issue, 152, 154
Patients, sexual abuse of, 47
Patient-therapist interaction, early psychotherapy studies on, 56–58
Peer supervision, 95, 179
Persecutory anxiety, defenses against, 57
Praise, distinguishing, from validation, 171–172
Privacy
  versus disclosure in psychotherapy supervision, 211–229
  disclosures, 222–228
  theoretical and developmental underpinnings, 217–222
  value of, in psychotherapy, 17–18
Process notes
  comparing discrepancy between recording and, 214
  in family therapy supervision, 123–124
Projective denigration, 69
Pseudogroup psychotherapy, 113–114
Psychiatric inpatient service

assignment of beginning
resident to, 75–77
responses of residents to
beginning work on,
77–78
Psychiatric resident
background of, 75–76
experiences of, during
supervision, 85–97
to psychiatric inpatient
service, 75–77
responses of, to beginning
work on psychiatric
service, 77–78
and separation anxiety, 147
skills needed by beginning, 75
supervision of beginning,
73–84
initial phase in, 78–79
suggested general
principles, 79–83
tasks of, 76–77
Psychiatric thinking, pendulum
of, 1
Psychodynamic group
psychotherapy, role of
therapist in, 102
Psychodynamic life narrative in
dealing with
emergency/crisis
states, 155–157
Psychosis, supervision of
patients with recurrent,
135–148
control versus
understanding, 139–141
cotherapy in, 143–144

countertransference reactions
in, 140–141
delusions in, 141
family concerns in, 142–143
hospitalization of patient in,
145–146
importance of reliability in,
139
issues of therapeutic frame
in, 138, 139
mirroring transference and
countertransference,
144–145
need for hospitalization of,
145–146
optimal therapeutic distance
for, 138–139
person versus case in,
137–139
quality time in, 136
and separation anxiety, 147
subjective meaning in
therapy, 141–142
suicide of patient in, 146–147
Psychotherapy
early studies of
patient-therapist
interaction, 56–58
education of students in, 1–2
as essential, 1
redefining to emphasis
person versus case,
137–139
training components of, 99
value of confidentiality and
privacy in, 17–18
waning of dynamic, 22–24

Psychotherapy students,
    education of, 1–2
Psychotherapy supervision. *See
    also* Cognitive-behavioral
    model; Emergency/crisis
    psychotherapy supervision;
    Ethical issues in psycho-
    therapy supervision; Family
    therapy supervision; Group
    therapy supervision
analytic training in, 15
beginning psychiatric
    resident in, 73–84
boundaries in, 96
clinical attitude in, 96–97
of clinical work, 99
closed-door model of, 17–22
cultural issues in, 53–55
    definition of culture in, 55
    dimensions of, in Canada
        and United States,
        63–65
    early studies of
        patient-therapist
        interaction, 56–58
    impact of cultural
        differences, 60–61
    professional
        underrepresentation
        of cultural groups,
        64–65
    psychotherapy training,
        58–60
    sense of self in, 61–62
definition of emergency and
    crisis in, 151
dual relationship in, 15–17, 31

ethical issues in, 11–36
failures in
    capacity of knowledge,
        256–257
    latent aspects of, 250–251
    manifest, 234–236
    paradigms of
        psychotherapy,
        251–254
    parallelism, 246–249
    rapport and good enough,
        236–246
    supervisory infallibility,
        231–234
gender issues in
    communication, 41–43
    consenting adults in, 46–47
    impact of gender on
        communication, 41–43
    need to identify with
        supervisor, 45–46
    recommendations in, 49–50
    in resident selection and
        evaluation of
        supervisors, 47–49
    and sexual abuse of
        patients, 47
    sexual embarrassment in,
        47
    supervisor-trainee
        boundaries in, 43–44
    supervisor-trainee
        competitiveness in,
        44–45
goal of, 73, 85–86
Hungarian method of, 14–15,
    16

identity crisis in, 22–24, 23
initial phase of, 78–79
as interactive learning
    process, 53–54
joint patient interviews in,
    81–82
language in, 65–69
latent aspects of failure in,
    250–251
legal issues in, 11–14, 23–27,
    24–27
literature on ethics of, 29–31
multifaceted nature of
    relationship with
    resident, 8–10
negligence as issue in,
    25–26
peer, 95, 179
as personal undertaking, 2
privacy versus disclosure in,
    211–229
  nondisclosures, 222–228
  theoretical and
      developmental
      underpinnings,
      217–222
rapport in, 95–96
regulation and oversight in,
    13
and sexual abuse of patients,
    47
suggested general principles
    in, 79–83
supervisee's experience in,
    85–97
supervision or therapy in,
    14–17

tasks of resident on inpatient
    service, 76–77
third-party payment for, 13
Psychotherapy supervisor
  development of, 189–207
    characteristics of, 196–197
    communication, 202
    dissolution of dyad,
        202–203
    history, 190–191
    intrapsychic, 199–201
    objectives of, 191–195
    research, 198
    status and roles of,
        201–202
    technique of, 195–196
    training for supervisors,
        203–207
    transference-like factors,
        199–201
  fiduciary obligation of, 31–36
  functions of, 87–90
  gender in evaluation of,
      47–49
  identifying characteristics of,
      86–87
  infallibility of, 231–234
  interactions in job, 90–97
  linear, 93
  need to identify with, 45–46
  paradigm of, 12, 14
  and recommendation of
      publications, 4
  relationship between
      supervisee and, 2–3
  as role model, 5–8, 18–20
  standard of care for, 27–29

Psychotherapy supervisor
  (continued)
  transmission of information
    in, 3–8
  triangular, 93–94, **94**
Psychotic patient. *See* Psychosis
Punishment, superiority of
    reinforcement over, 178–179

Rapport
  establishing in
    supervisor-resident
    relationship, 90–91,
    95–96
  and good enough
    supervision, 236–246
Reinforcement, superiority of,
    over punishment, 178–179
Resident selection, gender in,
    47–49
Response acquisition
    procedures in
    cognitive-behavioral model
    of supervision, 174–175
Response disinhibition
    procedures in
    cognitive-behavioral model
    of supervision, 176–178
Response inhibition procedures
    in cognitive-behavioral
    model of supervision,
    178–179
Response shaping and
    strengthening procedures in
    cognitive-behavioral model
    of supervision, 175–176
Rogers, Carl, 16, 19

Role-playing
  in development of
    psychotherapy
    supervisor, 196
  in family therapy
    supervision, 127
Roy v. Hartogs, 32

Scapegoating, 69, 102–103
Schizophrenia. *See* Psychosis,
    supervision of patients with
    recurrent
Self-disclosure, 220–221
Self-experiences, 222
Self-exposure, 220
Self-help groups, 23
Self psychology, shame in,
    218–219
Separation anxiety, 147
Sex incongruence, advantages
    to, in supervision, 46
Sexual abuse of patients, 47
Sexual harassment, 34–35
Shame, 218–219
Simmons v. United States,
    25–26
Simulation in family therapy
    supervision, 127
Skills training in
    cognitive-behavioral model
    of supervision, 173
  response acquisition
    procedures, 174–175
  response disinhibition
    procedures, 176–178
  response inhibition
    procedures, 178–179

response shaping and strengthening procedures, 175–176

Solution focused therapy, 121

Sorcerer's Apprentice phenomenon, 77

Standard of care for psychotherapy supervisors, 27–29

Strategic techniques, 122

Structural therapy, 122

Subgrouping, 102–103

Suicide of psychotic patient, 146–147

Supervision group, 113–115

Supervisory problem solving in cognitive-behavioral model of supervision, 172–173

Supervisory reinforcement, 176

Systems theory, 122, 123

Talking therapy, 78

Tarasoff v. Regents of the University of California, 26–27

Termination of psychotic patient, 147

Therapy, breaking parameters of, 225–226

Third-party payment for psychotherapy supervision, 13

Trainee, need of, to identify with supervisor, 45–46

Training for psychotherapy supervisors, 203–207

Transference
in family therapy supervision, 128. *See also* Countertransference
mirroring of psychotic patient, 144–145

Treatment of the therapist, 180

Triadic supervision, 112–113

Triangular supervision, 93–94

Tripartite model of human functioning, 168

Unit director, importance of, in setting educational mission, 76

United States, dimensions of cultural experience in, 63–64

Validation strategies, 170–172

Videotapes
in closed-door model of supervision, 17–22
and development of psychotherapy supervisor, 196
in family therapy supervision, 124
and supervisee's experience of supervision, 95

Viennese Psychoanalytic Institute, 190

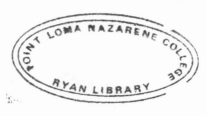